THE LUSH LONG HAIR CARE GUIDE

Over 50 Tips & Ideas to longer, healthier hair

Third Edition

ALLISON TYSON

Before you start your journey to longer luscious hair, take a photo* of your hair.

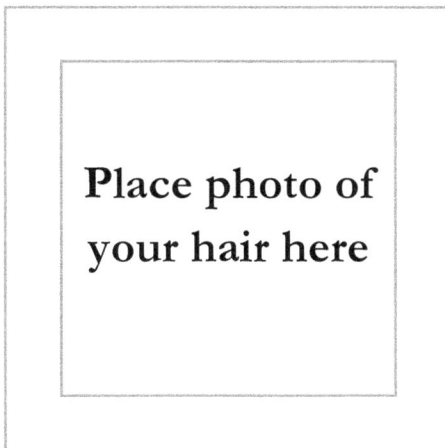

```
Place photo of
your hair here
```

*Back of the head shots are best

Hair Journey Start Date:

Goal Length:

Describe your hair:

Disclaimer

All material within this publication is for information purposes only.

This book is not intended to be a substitute for taking proper medical advice and should not be relied upon in this way. The author cannot accept any responsibility for illness arising from the failure to seek professional medical advice.

The information contained herein is not intended to cover all possible uses, directions, precautions, warnings, drug interactions, allergic reactions or adverse effects. If you have questions about the recommendations suggested, please seek professional advice from your doctor, pharmacist or health provider before commencing any treatments.

CONTENTS

Raising the dead

Has your crowning glory become a dreaded rat's nest? Are you doing one hair treatment after the other, looking for the next miracle cure? Tired of the same disappointing outcome?

Well, join the club! Millions of people all over the world, including myself, are looking for cures to their hair woes.

Prior to having my two kids, my hair care regime included benign neglect and indifference. It was only when my once luscious locks began to stick together like Velcro® and I appeared to have half the hair I used to, that my hair finally got my attention. In an endeavour to rid my hair of those dreadful 'bad hair days' I started clutching at miracle cures, quick fixes and some not so inexpensive solutions. Making little headway and with limited success, who was I kidding? It just kept getting worse! As the shedding increased and the width of my ponytail decreased, frustration set in. So, like a dog with a bone I went looking for answers.

The outcome of this book resulted from a three prong attack that included investigating medical research, folklore and hidden truths behind some outlandish claims.

After scouring the internet, partaking in online polls, stalking the forums and haunting the chat rooms, I found it! A wealth of valuable, economical and nature-friendly answers that I am going to share with you! Tips and Ideas that have brought my hair back to life.

Before I reveal to you over 50 Tips & Ideas to salvage your hair we need to establish some facts.

1

(If you are the sort of person who secretly reads the end of a novel first and can't wait to get started; in **Appendix- I** of this book I have included a quick reference summary of Tips & Ideas and **Appendix – II** contains the cheat sheet of stuff to try, buy, do and avoid. Otherwise, stick around and read what I found !)

Getting our facts straight

Fact 1: Hair is dead

Unlike our skin which is alive, hair is made up of dead cells, keratin and water. Hair cannot heal the damage we may unknowingly or deliberately be inflicting upon it.

Sad but also true, you only get one chance with your hair. The short term benefits of torturing your hair into submission for a night out can come at the cost of damaging the entire structure of your precious mane. Once you've inflicted damage, you can't permanently repair it. Your weakened hair becomes increasingly easier to damage and your current hair-care practices, or lack of, could be exacerbating and compounding further damage.

This is why it is so important to treat and pamper your luscious locks, to prevent damage in the first place. It's the reason you've chosen to read this book!

One essential part of preventing damage is to adopt a good hair care routine.

Regular Care --> The Hair You Deserve.

Fact 2: Hair is like an onion: it has many layers

Your hair shaft is composed of three distinct parts from outside to inside: *cuticle, cortex* and *medulla*.

The *cuticle* is the hard shingle-like outer layer of your hair shaft composed of overlapping, transparent, scale-like cells. This scale-like armour protects the more fragile core (cortex and medulla) of the hair fibre.

An undamaged healthy *cuticle* lies flat along the strand's surface, giving hair a shiny, smooth appearance that won't tangle because there is nothing for it to snag against.

Stress, poor diet, lack of sleep, excessive heat, hairstyling and other friction, as well as excessive exposure to nature's elements: sun, wind and water, can degrade the protective abilities of the *cuticle*.

Over time the *cuticle's* shingles lift, making hair feel rough, dull looking and increasingly difficult to manage. When the *cuticle* can no longer keep the inner hair fibre components tightly wrapped, split ends occur and the fibres begin to fray, causing breakage.

The *cortex* takes up most of the room in the hair shaft. It contains the pigment that gives your hair its natural colour and is responsible for giving your hair its strength and elasticity.

When your hair is chemically dyed, permed, relaxed or straightened, it is the *cortex* layer that is permanently affected, seldom to your hair's benefit.

The *medulla*, also called the marrow of the hair, is usually only found in coarse, thick hair. It is a hollow shaft found inside the *cortex*. Fine and naturally blonde hair is often lacking a *medulla*, and is more susceptible to damage. With no 'backbone', fine and thin hair cannot sustain the persistent torture we inflict on it like our thicker, coarser-haired friends.

Fact 3: The circle of life

Hair goes through a natural growth cycle throughout our lives, which is dictated by genetics. Genetics also determine the number of hairs on your head and the diameter of each of these hairs.

For most of us, at any given time, the majority of hair fibres are actively growing (anagen phase), while a small number of hair follicles stop growing and prepare to shed (catagen) or take a break (telogen phase).

With increasing age, your health and genetics, the number of hair follicles that go on a break (as mentioned above) increases, which can lead to noticeably thinner-looking hair.

Each of these facts is imperative to understanding how your hair grows and what hair is made of. Each of these facts can be manipulated in your favour to enable you to grow lusher, longer, healthier hair in a faster amount of time.

So, how do you maintain your crowning glory and get growing????

Let's get to it!

Going coconuts

The best way to keep damage to a minimum is to condition your hair regularly from root to tip, inside and out. Regular conditioning helps your hair to keep the cuticle intact, reduces friction, adds shine and lessens the static charge on your hair. This is common knowledge. But contrary to what you may already know, not many products actually penetrate into your hair shaft to give it the thorough conditioning it needs.

My number one recommendation as a hair conditioner is Coconut oil.

The Facts: Coconut Oil can pass between the cuticle's protective shingles and is easily absorbed by the cortex. It's a wonderful natural solution to keeping the scalp healthy and promotes healthy hair and growth.

The critical difference between coconut oil and other oils, including synthetic and fragrant mixes, is that coconut oil penetrates through the hair cuticle and reaches the cortex.[1] The low molecular weight of coconut oil allows it to be easily absorbed through your hair's layers.[2] So, unlike many topical creams and lotions, coconut oil is absorbed into the hair shaft and will not simply sit 'on' your hair making it heavy, dull and more prone to oiliness.[2]

Studies have established coconut oil has protective effects and the ability to actually help make hair stronger. For example, presoaking hair with coconut oil before using harsh chemicals, like bleach, will soften the effects and damage these agents can have on your hair.

Coconut oil is best used as a pre-shampoo conditioning treatment, or blended with shop-bought shampoos. This procedure will protect the hair from being stripped of its natural oils during the shampooing process. I'll discuss the effects of shampoo later in the book.

Not all oils are created equal

Whist studies have proven that coconut oil is one of the best oils for your hair, there are other oils you can experiment with that will help protect your tresses and make them softer and more manageable.

Olive and avocado oil have the ability to penetrate all the way into the hair shaft, although not to the extent that coconut oil does.[2]

Sweet almond oil, mineral oil and jojoba oil smooth the hair cuticle and cut down on friction but do not penetrate into the hair shaft. Massaging with these oils can add shine and lustre to your hair.

Each of these oils can be found in current hair care products but most are unfortunately mixed with synthetic formulas or are in such minute amounts that they compromise their ability to help your hair.

The arrogant oil

Argan oil is loved for the shine and lustre it can give, without the oily residue that heavier oils like coconut and olive oil can leave on fine hair. Its only drawback is that it is expensive when compared to readily available olive, coconut, and even jojoba oil.

A superior oil that comes at a superior price that should be used sparingly for best results.

The Facts: Argan oil, otherwise known as Moroccan oil, is exceptionally rich in fatty acids, antioxidants and vitamin E.[3] This makes it very useful in restoring, renewing and repairing the damage to hair caused by destructive factors like heat, over styling and chemical processing.

Rich in omega 3 fatty acids, Argan oil strengthens the protein bonds in hair and improves hair's strength. Being very similar in composition to olive oil,[4] Argan oil also easily penetrates into the follicles and enhances the elasticity of your hair. Argan oil is very nourishing for the growth of hair when used in conjunction with scalp massages, as it regulates sebum production and reduces inflammation.[4]

A sticky subject

Castor oil is regularly touted as a hair growth stimulant. It is a natural, ancient Indian remedy for thinning hair. When applied regularly to the scalp, three times a week, it is believed to help hair to grow healthier, thicker and for some, faster.

The Facts: The natural antifungal and antibacterial properties of castor oil protect your scalp from infections, like dandruff and fungus, which can cause some forms of hair loss.[5]

Castor oil also cleanses the scalp by removing dirt and bacteria, whilst it's healing properties can cure scalp infections. As a natural emollient castor oil can prevent hair from becoming brittle by hydrating and moisturising your hair shaft and scalp. These attributes have enabled castor oil to become renowned throughout India for its hair growth qualities.

Be aware that castor oil can darken hair and is quite viscous, so it must be blended with a carrier oil, not used as an everyday conditioning treatment.

Chemical warfare on your hair

For the two decades that I was dying and torturing my hair, I was blissfully unaware of the actual damage I was inflicting. Brittle hair and split ends were an acceptable norm. My quick fixes and expensive salon visits were just a bandaid to the underlying growing number of my hair problems. You see, like many of us, I did not fully understand that chemical damage occurs <u>every time</u> you colour, perm, relax and straighten your hair.

I acknowledge there are those amongst us who will continue to dye and chemically alter their hair. Reading the boxes and being aware of what you are putting onto your hair will help lessen damage. Don't always believe the hype; the front of the box and TV commercials will tell you one story, whereas the actual ingredients will tell you another.

The Facts: Synthetic hair dyes penetrate into the cortex of the hair, binding to and altering your natural pigment. For the chemicals to penetrate into the cortex, the cuticle of the hair needs to be lifted (remember those protective overlapping scale-like cells we mentioned at the start of the book?). That's why ammonia and hydrogen peroxide, or a bleaching solution, is used in synthetic hair dye. The ammonia and peroxide break down parts of the keratin (the protein hair is made from) in your hair each time you colour and can raise your hair's pH to damaging levels.

The lifting of the cuticle causes weathering of the hair; some cuticles are destroyed and some will not close properly after repeated colouring. The more weathered the cuticle, the rougher your hair will feel, and the more it will look like the proverbial 'rat's nest' you see on some people with long hair that has been coloured repeatedly over time. Chemical colouring removes keratin and eventually weakens your hair to the point that it breaks off. Colouring a cuticle that has not fully closed will mean an accelerated loss of pigment. This means you will have to re-dye your hair more often.

Some chemical dye companies claim their product helps repair the hair or make it feel fuller. However, if the product contains peroxide or ammonia, it is still going to damage your hair.[6] The volumising effect of the hair-colouring process will not make your hair fibres thicker, but can make hair fibres rougher, creating the appearance and feel of thicker hair. This is because the rougher texture causes neighbouring hair fibres to 'grip' each other, rather than slide past each other the way smooth fibres do, leading to increased friction and the more likelihood of hair snagging and snapping.

Permanent waving (the perm) and chemical straightening or relaxers use chemicals to disrupt the cortex's internal structure and change the hair's outward appearance. In order to change the shape of the hair, chemicals break the bonds that give the hair its structure by penetrating the cuticle and get into the cortex where they have their effect. The hair is then put into its new shape and 'neutralised' with further chemicals to ensure the new bonds stay in their new shape or hairstyle.

Colour you won't need to dye for

The only time I have ever grown my hair to my waist was when I was consistently using Henna. Contrary to popular belief it did not dry out my hair, cause split ends or fade.

The Facts: Henna does not lift the cuticle of the hair the way chemical hair colours do, nor will it break down the protein structure of hair or cause cancer. [63] When you colour with henna, your hair shaft is coated and the hair is stained to a desired colour.[7] See Idea 2 in **Appendix – I** for the various shades, not just red, of henna.

Henna also penetrates the cuticle layer through to the cortex; however it does not affect the structure of your hair in a negative way, like chemical colouring does. As the henna bonds with your hair's keratin proteins, it makes your hair more resistant to breakage and stronger. As it also contains hennotannic acid, a natural astringent, your scalp surface is tightened and the follicles strengthen their grasp on the hairs, lessening accidental shedding from overzealous brushing and styling.[8]

Colouring your hair with henna gives you the benefit of enhancing your natural colour, covering grey hairs and enhancing hair with natural looking highlights. Unfortunately, some companies add chemical dyes to their henna mixes. If the box has numbers listed in the ingredients, put it down and walk away.

Dying from the inside out

Just about everyone likes to experiment with bleaching their hair during their lifetime. The results can vary depending on your starting colour and hair type. Getting the look and feel of fairy-floss can easily be achieved overnight, as can unflattering tones of burnt orange with white roots if left in the hands of the inexperienced.

Dark hair-> Expectations that defy logic-> Bottle of bleach->Epic hair failure

The Facts: Like chemical dyes, bleaching your hair (also called decolourizing) changes hair structure to give you a new hair colour. The process involves the use of a 'developer' or 'activator' (usually hydrogen peroxide) to soften and raise the cuticle of the hair to allow bleaching of the underlying pigment cells in the cortex. This chemical process can severely weaken the structure of your hair shaft.

Unlike dying your hair, instead of depositing a colour into the hair shaft, the bleaching agent penetrates the shaft and disperses the colour molecules that are already there. The more colour molecules that are dispersed, the lighter the hair becomes. This chemical treatment can be especially damaging to hair by depleting essential proteins,[6] and can cause the hair to become brittle and fragile.

Relax - don't do it

Contrary to what you may have been told through extensive marketing campaigns, chemically altered pin-straight hair takes a lot of work and over time the treatments can take their toll on the health of your hair and wallet, I found this out the hard way. Just like the perms for curls, permanent straightening of hair changes the internal structure of your hair causing damage.

The Facts: Relaxed hair has been a popular ritual in the African-American culture for decades. The process was developed for people with coarse, wiry, curly hair, who wanted more manageable, 'straighter' hair.

Nowadays, relaxed hair is popular in mainstream society, and is commonly referred to as chemical straightening. Usually, chemical straightening is marketed as a solution to tame frizz and to provide pin-straight hair to those of us with kinks and curls.

Relaxed hair and chemical straightening change the basic structure of the hair shaft. The chemicals penetrate the cortex and loosen the natural curl pattern. Once this process is performed, it is irreversible. Whilst the desired effect is silky straight hair, the process leaves the hair weak and extremely susceptible to breakage and further damage. The chemicals do not help the hair, they strip it of its natural strength and elasticity. Research studies have also linked exposure to phthalates and other endocrine-disrupting chemicals to uterine and endometrial cancer. [61]

Recently, keratin smoothing treatments which promise to replenish, straighten and protect hair without nasty chemicals have come under fire.[9] Heated debates have focused on the safety of formaldehyde and related carcinogenic chemicals in supposedly benign ingredients. Even the 'formaldehyde-free' versions have been found to still contain formaldehyde.[10]

Different brush strokes for different folks

Look down at the bathroom sink or floor after your next over zealous brushing episode. If you are finding what looks like the hairs from a heavily malting animal, you may need to change the way you brush your hair.

The Facts: There are two camps when it comes to the art of brushing your hair. One theory attests to brushing hair to stimulate the scalp and distribute the hair's sebum. Sebum protects your hair and scalp as it travels naturally down the hair shaft, thus giving your hair moisture and shine, and stops it from drying out. Manual brushing moves the oil from the scalp through to the hair's length and ends, nourishing these parts of the hair.[11]

The alternative view is that overzealous brushing is a major contributor to hair damage, causing breakage and hair loss. If you are using the wrong type of brush, what is known as cuticle chipping can result from the abrasion of your hair against the brush's bristle.[2] Cuticle chipping weakens the hairs protective armour leading to hair that is susceptible to breakage. In some cases when the brush hits a snag, it can pull hair to breaking point or rip it out from the roots. The follicle that attaches the hair to the scalp is like a glove surrounding the living part of the hair strand. The constant tugging from harsh brushing pulls the hair out of your scalp.

Brushing wet hair is always a huge no no. When hair is wet it swells, and in this state it is very fragile and therefore it's easier for

15

hair breakage to occur. If you choose to brush, wait for your hair to dry first.[2]

It's not nice to tease

Back-brushing, back-combing or teasing your hair are some of the most damaging forms of aggressive torture you can inflict on your precious tresses. The negative effects can build up over time and become visible broken, spikey, little hairs that sit at the top of your head and won't lie down. Remember those '80's soft Metal Bands?

The Facts: These techniques are extremely harmful[12] because they require the scales of the cuticle, which all lie pointing towards the tip of the shaft like tiles on a roof, to be lifted in the opposite direction. The cuticle scales are easily ripped off the next time a brush passes over them. There is no way to repair this damage which leads to weakened hair that snaps off easily.

Plastics aren't always fantastic

Experimenting with the type of brush and/or comb you are using will give you an indication if you are causing hair damage. Again, comb and brush over a bathroom sink to check for broken hairs.

The Facts: Often plastic combs have a thin seam on the tips of the teeth. Hair can catch and break on these rough and sometimes sharp seams. In some cases, combing with a plastic comb can build up a static charge, which can result in frizz.

Long hair specialists often recommend 100% pure boar bristle brushes with wooden bases to prevent the build-up of static electricity during brushing, and because the bristles on the brush are the closest to replicating the natural structure of hair.[11] Avoid brushes with plastic nibs on the ends of the bristles as these can snag on your fragile hair.

A quality comb is smooth without any areas that could damage hair.

It's all in the hands

When it comes to combing and detangling fragile hair, you can't go past the very effective use of finger combing and wide tooth combs, especially if you have curly hair. Never underestimate the damage over-enthusiastic brushing and combing can have, especially on wet and tangled hair.[6]

Avoiding the chop

If you really want longer hair, stop cutting it! It really is that easy.

Logic will tell you that if your hair is growing 1cm a month, but you are cutting 1cm off every four weeks, you will see no difference in the length of your hair. You may see an increase in thickness, but the length will not change because you are cutting your hair at the same rate it is growing.

Unfortunately, most of us have some type of damage to our hair, and cutting it is the only way to get rid of this damage.

The Facts: Damaged hair breeds tangles and thus splits and breakage. Hair that is damaged is also rougher and the frayed ends snag more easily. The constant breakage will limit your hair's maximum length, regardless of how fast your hair grows.

If you have healthy hair that you want to grow long, trim it only once or twice a year. But if your hair is damaged, you need to trim it more often to reap the benefits and keep damage to a minimum. Alternatively, you could cut all the damaged length off and start again.

String theory

Picture your damaged hair as a piece of string. The end of that string is frayed and starting to unravel. No matter where you cut, the ends are going to start to fray and unravel. String unravels at the same rate regardless of whether you cut 1cm from the end, or 3cm from the end. The same applies to your hair.

The Facts: Frequent micro-trims for damaged hair are what you need to help minimise damaged ends. Dustings (or micro-trimming) refers to a trim that is so slight (1/2cm), the pieces left on the floor look like dust. Dustings will ensure the ends of your hair stay as intact as possible, resulting in less breakage and not too much length will be lost at the one time. Micro-trims also benefit the slower growing hairs by allowing them to 'catch up' to your faster growing hairs.

Fancy that: there is some truth to the myth that cutting hair makes it grows faster! It's just breaking off less.

Friend or foe

There's a biblical story about a man named Samson and his lover Delilah. Samson was very strong and had exceptionally long hair. The tale tells of Delilah tricking Samson into having all his hair cut off. As a result he lost his strength and power.

Like Samson, many of us find ourselves suddenly rendered powerless and agreeing to ideas we normally wouldn't when we sit in the hairdresser's chair to have our hair cut.

Sitting mute and pretending to read the out-of-date women's magazines whilst the hairdresser's scissors glide through your precious hair, whilst in your minds eye calculating how long it is going to take to grow your hair back...this time, is not the way to achieve your hair goals.

The Facts: Finding a good hairdresser who knows how to listen is a must if you want to grow lush healthy hair. You'll need one that understands you are trying to grow your hair and knows how to micro-trim not style cut. Hairdressers need your input if they are to cut your hair the way you want it cut. There are some hairdressers who consider their work a form of art and you their canvas. If you are trying to grow your hair long and healthy, avoid these types of hairdressers as they will not listen and you will leave the salon disappointed every time.

If you have been a victim of a seriously bad salon experience, you may decide to avoid hairdressers altogether and cut your hair yourself. If you choose to do so, make sure you use a pair of very sharp hairdressing scissors. Blunt scissors can wreak havoc on your ends and actually cause more split ends.[12]

Water - the elixir of life

Water is essential for proper hair growth. Eight to ten glasses of water a day are often recommended. Just by drinking water you can increase the amount of moisture in your hair.

The Facts: Water comprises approximately one quarter of the weight of a strand of hair. When hair has the proper amount of water, it will respond by being supple and shiny. Hair deprived of its adequate daily water requirements may stop growing completely.

Water flushes the internal system, eliminates toxins and keeps you hydrated. Water is also vital for the function of every cell in your body, including hair follicles which are nourished by water and blood from inside the body.

If your hair roots are deficient in adequate water levels, your locks will eventually become dry and brittle. When the body is dehydrated, circulation to the base of the outer skin, the scalp and hair roots may shut down as an emergency measure so that more water is not lost through evaporation from the skin's surface.

Sealed with a rinse

A blast of cold water at the end of your shower is a sure way to wake you up in the morning and give your hair a frizz free start to the day. It is believed hot water opens the hair cuticles and thirty seconds under cold water will close the cuticles. With the cuticle closed moisture is trapped within the hair, creating softer, silkier and shinier hair.

The Facts: Hydrotherapy uses hot and cold water rinses to stimulate blood circulation. Hot water draws blood flow to the epidermis; cold water exerts the opposite effect and encourages blood to retreat from the surface to the body's organs.[13] Alternating between hot and cold water during your regular shower routine leads to better circulation to the scalp; more nutrients are delivered to the hair roots, leading to better hair growth.

Cold water also constricts the opening of the sebaceous glands to help moderate sebum production on the scalp.

What's in the water?

Showering using hard water, which has a high mineral content, can cause build-up on the hair shaft, leading to dull, lifeless and hard to brush hair.

The Facts: There are several water contaminants that can cause hair to fall out or illnesses that contribute to hair loss.

Selenium:

Generally occurs in the food we eat as a trace mineral, however it is also an element found in ores. Most commonly, this element can reach toxic levels when it gets into the water system from the run-off from refineries and mines. Excessive overdosing of selenium can lead to hair loss.

Mercury:

Found in fish and polluted waterways.

Lead:

Water travelling from old lead pipes to the shower may be a prescription for hair loss from lead posioning.

Zinc:

Food naturally contains trace amounts of zinc, which is an essential nutrient needed by our bodies. Contamination occurs when there are excessive amounts of zinc in the water caused by such things as metal manufacturing industries and electrical utilities.

Aluminium:

In water it can cause health problems such as anemia which in turn leads to hair loss.

Arsenic and thallium:

Can cause hair to fall out and make you very sick.

Copper:

Protein damage to hair can be significantly eliminated by removing copper from the water supply.[12]

Swim protection

Growing up it was easy to tell which kids attended regular swim classes or were serious swimmers. They either had green hair or hair so stiff it felt like cardboard. Without rinsing hair after a morning session with my swim coach, my hair would dry into stiffened ponytails that would feel and 'crunch' just like straw. Swimming can be great for your fitness, but a nightmare for your hair.

The Facts: Chlorine from swimming pools can destroy much-needed proteins in our hair. Depleted of protein, hair can become very dry and brittle. Blonde and grey hair has been known to turn green because of exposure to chlorine pools.

Some hairdressers and hair extension companies recommend club soda as a rinse after swimming to neutralise the effects of chlorine. The carbonation helps break up the mineral deposits and rinses the chlorine effectively from your hair.

Chelating shampoos will also remove chlorine. Most work by using a chemical called ethylenediaminetetraacetic acid (EDTA), which binds to the chlorine and removes it from the hair. However, these shampoos can be harsh on your hair with repetitive use, as EDTA is also an active ingredient in laundry detergents and cleaners.[14]

As well as chlorine, salt water from the beach and swimming pools can also have devastating effects on your hair. The salt water lifts the hair cuticle, and moisture is lost from within. This can cause a dry, rougher-than-usual hair texture, commonly referred to in the beauty industry as beach waves/curls.

Pooh pooh the shampoo?

We are taught from an early age to shampoo our hair to keep it "squeaky" clean. However, shampooing may be causing more damage than we realise.

The Facts: Most shampoos available contain harsh, drying concoctions that are extremely damaging to our hair by stripping it of its natural oils (sebum) and can cause cancer. [62] Also, with each shampoo, these chemicals (especially sodium laureth sulphate) can cause protein loss to the hair shaft.[6] Over time, this protein loss reduces the diameter of the hair shaft and creates thinner, weaker hair.

The main culprits in these shampoos are:

- ammonium laureth sulphate
- ammonium lauryl sulphate
- sodium laureth sulphate (SLS)
- sodium lauryl sulphate

New formulas are created every year, so be on the lookout and try to avoid any shampoos that contain ingredients with mixes that include the words sodium, lauryl/laureth, ammonium and sulphate/sulphide.

Both sodium lauryl sulphate and sodium laureth sulphate are used as detergents and wetting agents in car wash soaps, engine degreasers and garage floor cleaners. These chemicals are present in 90 percent of shampoos that create foam or lather. Damaged hair is more susceptible to SLS protein loss than undamaged hair containing an intact cuticle.[6]

Propylene glycol is found in most shampoos to give your shampoo its 'glide' and to maintain shelf life. It's also the active compound in antifreeze,[15] so just imagine what it could be doing to your hair!

To overcome problems associated with shampoos, you could start following the 'pooh pooh' movement whereby shampoo is avoided altogether.

But many of us are oiling our hair to maintain healthy hair or have naturally oily hair, so going without shampoo may not be an option. Alternatives to regular, harsh shampoos may be the way to go; you just need to find what works for you. Refer to the suggested shampoo tips in the **Appendix – I.**

The style council

Styling products tend to be the lesser evil in the battle against our hair woes but are still considered damaging when used excessively.

The Facts: Many types of mousse, hair sprays and gels contain alcohol or other agents that can be very drying. While there are some reformulated styling agents out there, many still contain alcohol, which is a major factor in drying out already damaged hair.

When your hair starts to move with these products in it, or you try to brush them out, your hair shafts adhere to each other, and the cuticle's protective shingles are ripped off the strand. This causes irreparable damage.

Your damaged hair then becomes more unruly, and unfortunately you'll probably try to tame this unruly hair with more drying products.

Go natural

It's difficult not to get caught up in the paradox of believing that keratin treatments, products containing SLS, silicones and chemical treatments can help you achieve healthy hair, but how does this make sense? And who is really behind these outlandish claims anyway?

The Facts: So many hair products today expose your hair and scalp to harsh chemicals. As many of us move towards healthier lifestyles, we are drawn to products that are marketed as pure and natural in the hope to attain healthier hair. Unfortunately, many of these well-known products only contain minute amounts of the beneficial oils, proteins and herbs they claim to possess. New products hit the shelves every month with new claims and 'miracle' ingredients, but most (or all) of them still include substances that are contributing to damaging your hair in the first place.

To attain or retain luscious, long, healthy hair, avoiding or limiting the use of chemicals, products containing sulphates and silicone, as well as products with ingredients that end in -cone, -conol or –xane may be the answer.

The short-term use of silicones in hair products, such as conditioners, will make your hair look sleek and less frizzy, because they are designed to collect on damaged cuticles to keep them smooth and fill in fractures.[16] Over time, however, they coat the hair shaft and seal out moisture, causing it to become frizzy and straw-like, with less defined curl and lustre. Nearly every 'name brand' product contains silicones; have a look the next time you are browsing the aisles at your local supermarket. Pick up a bottle and check the ingredients for yourself.

(N.B Some manufacturers of hair products are starting to listen, product ingredients with silicones containing "PEG" are water soluble and won't build up.)

As mentioned in Pooh pooh the shampoo chapter, shampoos often contain the cleanser ammonium laurel sulphate which strips your hair of sebum and leaves your hair unprotected. Sulphate shampoos are normally used to remove silicones and waxes. In the long run these shampoos are very drying and harsh on your hair.

Most fragrance ingredients are synthetic chemical concoctions put together to create a pleasant smell, but do nothing to enhance your hair.

Clever marketing campaigns draw our attention to these products, but informed choices will benefit your hair.

Bringing back what was lost

Protein and deep conditioning treatments help rebuild or add moisture back into your hair. Understanding when your hair needs protein or conditioning is the key to maintaining healthy hair. But knowing which treatment to use, and when to use it, is crucial.

The Facts: Protein treatments strengthen the hair. They're used to replace some of the protein lost from hair that is regularly coloured, permed or bleached (remember the fairy floss?). As a general rule of thumb, if your hair feels mushy or overly elastic when wet, this is a sign that you need a protein treatment. But remember, nothing beats keeping protein where it should be in the first place; in the strands.

Dry, brittle hair that reminds you of straw or feels crunchy at the ends is calling out for a deep moisturising treatment. Avoid using protein treatments on brittle hair. Whilst they help rebuild the hair fibres, protein at this point is more likely to have a further drying effect.

Brittle hair will need conditioning with substances containing a high lipid content. The higher the lipid content (the more greasy and thick the emollient), the better and longer it works, but the messier and harder it is to wash out.

Shea butter is an excellent example; it is rich in vitamins A, E and F. Vitamin F consists of two essential fatty acids, linoleic acid and alpha-linoleic acid. These acids, which make up 85 to 90 percent of the total fatty acid in Shea butter,[17] hydrate and revitalise the hair and scalp, giving you luxuriously soft, healthy hair.

Burnt to a crisp

Like many women, I thought my straightener was my best friend. For nearly ten years I chose to ignore the large amount of hairs that fell to the floor each time I would use it. My hair looked sleek and shiny but over time it started to feel increasingly brittle. The penny dropped when looking at photos I realised I had only half the hair I used to. And why did it look like I had randomly hacked into it with a razor?

The Facts: Budget straighteners usually come with metal plates. Under a microscope, these plates look like sandpaper. They don't distribute heat evenly and the abrasive surface can cause damage to your hair.

Ceramic straighteners are microscopically smooth and distribute heat evenly. Though they may not feel like they are damaging your hair, when used on a regular basis they can also take a destructive toll on the structure of your hair and cause very noticeable problems.[18]

Here's why. The hot tongs of straighteners damage the outer layer of the hair fibre, leading to a dry, weathered look with strands that split and snap off easily. Trichologists (scientists who study hair and scalps) link overuse of hair straighteners to creating more frizz, setting up a 'straightener usage' cycle.

Any heat over 180 degrees Celsius damages the cuticles of the hair. The cuticle should lie flat, but repeated straightening causes a breakdown in the cuticle. The 'slates' start to lift and the rough, uneven surface exposes the cortex, allowing the fibres to unravel.

This starts as split ends, but can reach all the way up the hair, causing it to break off.

Tools of mass destruction

Our blow driers, curling irons, crimpers, thermal brushes and flat irons are wonderful heat styling tools if used sparingly. But when used every day with a combination of questionable hair practises, they can dry out hair and cause a lot of damage. The effects of heat styling are always temporary; therefore the norm is to use them frequently. It is the frequency of use with these styling tools that breaks down your hair's resilience making it more susceptible to damage.

The Facts: The water in your hair is what makes it flexible. The heat from these appliances damage your hair by reducing its water content, softening the keratin and creating a loss of cuticle.[19]

If they are used too hot, over 180 degrees Celsius, they can actually cause the water in your hair to boil and form tiny bubbles of steam inside the softened hair shaft and weaken it.[19] This is evidenced by little white dots seen midway up the hair shaft, that eventually cause longer pieces of the hair to snap off.

Too much blow drying can cause the cuticles to open so far that even the best conditioners will fail to close them properly again. If the cuticles protective layers are damaged too often, your hair loses its strength and integrity and breakage will occur.

Some like it hot

Water that is too hot has the tendency to open the cuticle layers of your hair. If you use hot water to wash your hair, you can scald your hair, much like the effect of a curling iron, and this can lead to dull hair and make it more dry and brittle.

On the flipside, heat can also have a positive effect on your hair when used for deep conditioning treatments. When the heat causes the hair to open, it allows the conditioning agent to penetrate deeply.

Sock it to ya!

We all have days when we become bored with our hair and are looking for a change. Sometimes it is fun to shake things up a bit without sabotaging our healthy hair care routine.

But did you know that socks can give you super easy and natural looking curls with absolutely no heat? This is especially good for those of us with fine or thin hair. Magic happens when the 'sock-bun' is removed, revealing voluminous, Hollywood curls naturally, and with NO HEAT. See **Appendix - I** for *How to Make a Sock Bun Idea*. The sock can also be used to 'bulk up' the size of your bun while you wait for your hair to thicken up.

Doobie or not doobie

For straighter hair without scorching heat try the hair doobie, otherwise known as hair wrapping or the Saran wrap. The doobie helps to keep your hair looking smooth and frizz free, naturally. It can also help cut down on the time it takes to 'do' your hair.

African and Latin American women with chemically relaxed hair have used the doobie for decades to keep their relaxed hair straight and to protect it when sleeping or working. See **Appendix - I** for *How to doobie your hair*.

Hang Loose

Super slick ponytails that pull your hair too tight may give you an instant facelift but they also place a lot of stress on your hair follicles, contribute to breakage and lead to painful headaches.

The Facts: Hair RSI (Repetitive Stress Injury) can occur from wearing your hair in the same tight hairstyle too often. The damage comes from repeated tension on the same spot, which causes your delicate hairs in that area to eventually weaken and break.

A condition known as traction alopecia occurs when tight hair elastics, hair extensions or tight braids cause excessive tension and breakage of the shaft along the hairline.

Wearing loose styles like braided buns, cinnamon buns and French braids may help prevent this problem.

The buffalo track

Parting your hair in the same place can cause what is called a 'buffalo track'; that is, a well worn 'track' which appears as a permanent parting of the hair. The most common is the centre part. It is not a look that suits all face shapes.

The Facts: Over time, this track tends to widen. Traction alopecia can exacerbate the parting and cause thinning of the exposed area. Regularly 'retraining' your hair to part different ways will lessen the width of your 'buffalo track' and enable you to wear different styles.

Daylight robbery

Everyday, unbeknownst to you, you could be robbing yourself of healthy hair and causing damage to your luscious locks.

The Facts: Seat belts, backpacks, handbag straps and even leaning against the back of a chair reading your emails can pull and snag your hair, leading to breakages.

Daytime hair protection is essential to stopping accidental breakage, and means wearing your hair up during the day to protect it.

Vital vitamins

If you've experienced sudden or unexplained hair thinning, it's good advice to see a health provider to determine the cause. Do not be surprised if you are informed that your diet lacks certain essential vitamins.

A blood test can provide crucial indicators for what essential nutrients (if any) are missing in your diet and your individual needs.

The Facts: The following vitamins are recognised for their beneficial effects on the hair follicles and are considered to be critical for healthy, luscious hair growth:

Vitamin A:

Helps create vibrant, shiny hair because it contributes to fat synthesis in hair follicles, thus playing a huge part in the production of sebum. However, an excessive intake of vitamin A can be toxic and lead to hair loss.

Vitamin B8 (Inositol):

Considered one of the key nutrients to spur hair growth and prevent balding. As an antioxidant, B8 has a protective effect on hair follicles.

Vitamin B3 (Niacin):

Helps increase circulation to the scalp, and thus increases oxygen and other vitamin transportation to the scalp and follicles.

Vitamin B5 (Panthenol):

Studies have shown that topically applied panthenol has the ability to thicken and repair damaged hair.[20] The relatively small molecular structure of B5 allows it to penetrate the hair shaft and to hold moisture within each hair follicle. Thus, your hair is provided with pliability from the inside and this gives lustre on the outside.

Vitamin B9 (Folic acid):

Studies have found that a diet deficient in folic acid can lead to baldness. A folate deficiency occurs if you do not get an adequate amount of folic acid in your diet and can lead to anaemia.[21]

Vitamin B7 (Biotin):

Known also as vitamin H, biotin is responsible for the creation of keratin in our bodies and hair. Biotin is essential for the absorption and utilization of nutrients and enables fats and amino acids from your food to be converted to keratin for healthy hair and nails.

Studies have shown biotin deficiencies can result in brittle hair and nails, and hair loss.[22]

Vitamin C:

Helping your body's absorption of iron, vitamin C is crucial to prevent anaemia, a condition that can result in hair shedding.

Vitamin C is also useful for the production of collagen, an essential building block for healthy hair.

Vitamin E

This vitamin stimulates circulation in the scalp and helps with oxygen absorption. Vitamin E can be taken internally or applied topically to the scalp. Research has shown that vitamin E inhibits the androgen phase of the hair cycle and can prevent hair loss and balding associated with male pattern hair loss.[23]

Because of its remarkable moisturizing properties[24], vitamin E can also be applied topically to hair. To apply, open a capsule of vitamin E and massage into your scalp.

Hello sunshine

Not spending enough time in the outdoors can lead to a vitamin D deficiency, which is always a possible factor contributing to hair loss. An easy solution to increase your sunlight exposure is to take a ten-minute (early morning or late afternoon) stroll in the sun once a day to get your daily dose of vitamin D.[25]

The Facts: Hair loss and rickets are the primary symptoms of a vitamin D deficiency, along with psoriasis or a flaky scalp.

Sun kisses

The bad news is, too much ultraviolet light from direct sunlight on the cuticle has a similar effect to that of bleach.

The Facts: Over-exposure to UV rays weakens the internal structure of the hair, resulting in hair breakage and loss. Eventually the keratin (protein) of the hair breaks down and results in a gradual weakening of hair, which leads to chronic dryness and loss of pigment.

The sun kissed effect shows up as light streaks in the hair, often referred to as sun-bleached hair.

Supplements for suppleness

Take-out, packaged food and convenience meals can sometimes lack the crucial nutrients we need to grow lush, healthy hair. The aisles of the chemist and supermarkets are teeming with multivitamins and supplements touting their benefits. My quest lead me to compile this list of supplements specifically needed to grow a healthy head of hair.

The Facts:

Calcium:

A lack of calcium can result in weaker, smaller hairs that are more prone to fall out. Certain types of shampoos decrease the amount of calcium in the hair, causing hair loss.[26]

Iron:

Iron fuels hair growth by increasing circulation to the scalp. Iron deficiency prevents full development of the hair follicle and causes your hair to become weak and fragile.[27]

Magnesium:

This nutrient has been shown to reduce inflammation of the hair follicle. An inflamed hair follicle shuts down hair production and can lead to baldness. By reducing inflammation around the hair follicles, regeneration of existing hairs and new growth can begin.

Manganese:

An essential trace element, manganese prevents slow hair growth as it helps your body to use other nutrients like thiamine, biotin and vitamin C.

L-Lysine:

An amino acid which will help with the uptake of iron.[27]

Zinc:

According to one research paper, patients who suffered hair loss after surgery were given zinc sulphate tablets to stop hair shedding. The study found that all patients stopped losing hair after taking the zinc supplements.[28]

Zinc helps build protein and assists with the absorption of copper and iron. Zinc also works alongside vitamin A, and a deficiency in either can lead to dry hair and oily skin. However, excessive consumption of zinc can result in nausea and stomach irritation.

Silica:

Another important nutrient for hair health, silica can slow hair loss and improve the condition of hair and nails.[29] Organic silica can also be added to shampoo to help prevent baldness, stimulate hair growth and increase hair strength.

Iodine:

Iodine is an essential trace element. The thyroid gland relies on iodine to make the hormones necessary for the growth of healthy hair, teeth and bones. When we are deficient in this nutrient, hair can become weak or fall out completely.

Selenium:

Selenium is an important mineral for the health of your scalp. A deficiency may inhibit your hair's ability to grow, resulting in an overall thinning of your tresses.

Sulphur methylsulfonylmethane (MSM):

Your hair is composed of proteins (keratin) embedded in a sulphur-rich matrix.[12] Sulphur plays an important role in the regeneration of our cells and the growth of hair.[30] Also known as the beauty mineral and commonly used in arthritis treatments, sulphur methylsulfonylmethane in its purest form can prevent and reverse hair loss and restore hair colour.

Potassium:

Sodium levels are regulated by your potassium intake. A potassium deficiency (hypokalaemia) can cause your hair to fall out. High levels of sodium from hypokalaemia can damage the hair follicles and prevent the necessary nutrients from reaching your hair.

Nuts about nuts

Skip this chapter if you are allergic to nuts.

For a long time nuts have been touted as bad guys full of fats that should be avoided when it came to eating healthy. What we now know is nuts are a powerhouse of essential minerals for hair growth.

The Facts: One of the important benefits of nuts is that they provide the body with proteins, zinc and good fats. Eating a handful of mixed nuts is probably the best way to reap the benefits they have to offer and to stave off hunger pangs in a healthy way that will help with your hair growth.

Almonds, cashew and pecans:

A great source of zinc.

Brazil nuts:

One of nature's best sources of selenium, which is an important mineral for the health of your scalp. Be careful to eat no more than two each day as eating more than a few on a regular basis can lead to a toxic dose of selenium poisoning.

Hazelnuts:

Hazelnut oil is the best known source for vitamin E and a good source of B vitamins, calcium and another beneficial acid, linoleic acid.

Hazelnuts also contain substantial amounts of iron, zinc, protein and potassium. One of the major health benefits of hazelnuts is that they are rich in folic acid. Ancient Greeks appear to have been well aware of the health benefits of hazelnuts and used them to stimulate hair growth in bald people.

Walnuts:

Walnuts contain biotin and alpha-linolenic acid, an Omega-3 fatty acid, which can help condition your hair. They are also an excellent source of zinc.

What goes in, will sprout out

As established earlier, your beautiful hair has to be nourished from within before it starts its journey.. The benefits of a healthy diet, a little sunshine and adequate exercise will greatly influence the condition of your hair.

The Facts: Your scalp, hair follicles and blood are all needed to create every lock of hair on your head. This is where your luscious, long, healthy hair growth starts its journey. Hair is a record of your diet and nutrition, which means the food you eat directly influences the state of your hair.

Healthy hair diet

We are being told all the time what to eat to lose weight and get healthy. Now there is an eating plan just for the sake of growing your hair.

Here is the 'low down' on the foods to eat that will give your hair the best possible start on it's journey out of your head. The healthy hair diet includes green leafy vegetables, tofu, legumes, lentils, beans, beef, seafood, whole-grain cereals, sprouts, peanut butter, nuts, Vegemite (yeast extract), poultry, eggs and low-fat dairy.

The Facts: Protein is one of your hair's key building blocks, and insufficient protein intake can lead to a decrease in your hair's diameter, making hair look less than healthy.

Protein stimulates growth and is important in rebuilding and strengthening the hair shaft. A recent study concluded that a well-balanced diet should contain a substantial amount of protein, from 15-25 % of your daily food intake, depending on age, gender, activity levels and medical conditions.[31] This is particularly true for folk looking to improve the state of their hair, as inadequate protein can increase the likelihood of weak and brittle hair.

Eat plenty of iron-rich foods, like liver (avoid if you are pregnant) and other organ meat, whole grain cereals, dark green leafy vegetables, eggs, dates and raisins.

Foods such as carrots, eggs, spinach, cabbage, squash, mustard, soy beans, peanuts and pine nuts are rich in vitamin A and iodine.

Foods high in omega-3 fatty acids, such as fish, plant and nut oils, are the primary dietary source of omega-3 fatty acids. Dry, brittle hair and dry, itchy skin, all respond to a diet rich in omega-3s. Flaxseed oil and salmon are good sources of these acids. If you don't get enough fatty acids, especially the essential ones, your body can't produce its own 'D' vitamins. This will result in a deficiency.

Dark green vegies: spinach, broccoli, and kale are an excellent source of vitamins A and C. Dark green vegetables also provide iron and calcium.

Eggs are one of the best protein sources you can find. They also contain sulphur, biotin and vitamin B-12, which are important beauty nutrients.

Acai berries contain more grams of protein than eggs, and also contain omega 3, 6 and 9 fatty acids. Acai has been credited with helping improve the look and texture of hair, skin and nails.

Whole grains, including whole-wheat bread and fortified, whole-grain breakfast cereals, provide a hair-healthy dose of zinc, iron and B vitamins, para-aminobenzoic Acid (PABA) and folic acid. All combine to help hair grow. PABA is found naturally in whole grains and yeast.

Shellfish, oysters, tahini and pumpkin seeds all contain the hair-boosting abilities of zinc.

Low-fat dairy products like skim milk, cottage cheese and yoghurt are great sources of calcium, an important mineral for hair growth. They also contain whey and casein, two high-quality protein sources.

Diet disaster

Low calorie eating plans and crash dieting can result in hair loss.

The Facts: Your hair's growth cycle can be impacted negatively if you are not eating enough of the 'good stuff'. Starving yourself can cause a higher than normal number of hair follicles to shed their hair fibres. Important nutrients for healthy hair that are missing in your diet can stunt your hair growth and lead to hair loss.

An apple a day

Apple cider vinegar (ACV) is a mild acid made from fermenting apples. For centuries, ACV has been credited for its abundant health benefits, such as dispersing minerals throughout your system and aiding digestion when taken internally.

The Facts: The acids and enzymes in ACV can kill the pathogens associated with alopecia.[32] When used on your scalp as a clarifying rinse, ACV's mild acidic properties help promote circulation, act as a natural antiseptic, dissolve excessive fatty deposits, reduce scaling of the scalp and unblock hair follicles to promote growth and slow hair loss.

ACV rinses also deter conditioner build up, help de-tangle your hair, balance pH and seal the cuticles to lessen frizz.

Go bananas!

Bananas are a super food when it comes to hair health, they seem to also make monkeys very happy too!

The Facts: Bananas have high concentrations of potassium which protects the inner and outer cells of your hair, prevent breakage, reduce hair loss and regulate hair growth.[33] Potassium also acts as a conditioner which allows your hair to stay manageable and strong. Banana applied topically to the hair is said to help repair and soothe damaged hair.[34]

Eating bananas is also one of the easiest ways to get tryptophan, an amino acid building block of protein. Bananas contain traces of zinc and B vitamins including B6 (pyridoxine) which influences hormone activity, sleep patterns and iron uptake.

Molasses

For centuries, some Chinese and Central American cultures have used molasses to stimulate hair growth.

The Facts: Molasses is a natural source of essential minerals, vitamins and trace elements. It can be taken internally to strengthen weak and thinning hair as it provides iron, calcium, potassium, phosphorous, copper and magnesium. In addition, blackstrap molasses is a good source of vitamin B6 and selenium.

In Jamaica, molasses is applied to the hair and left in all day, then washed out. Jamaicans have found that the molasses masque stops breakages, darkens hair, defines the natural colour, adds softness and gives hair a healthy sheen.

Rumour has it

Steadily gaining in popularity, delicious and nutritious Rooibos tea (*aspalathus linearis*), sometimes called redbush tea, is now available in many local supermarkets. Rooibos tea is drunk for its naturally high antioxidant content and pleasant taste. Not so well known are its effects on growing healthy hair.

The Facts: The native Rooibos plant is indigenous to South Africa and has been used for many centuries by the indigenous Khoisan tribes of the region. The rumour says that an anthropology professor studying different African tribes was impressed by the condition of the hair and skin of the Khoi compared to other tribes in the area.

The Khoisan used the leaves of the Rooibos bush to make herbal remedies for common ailments. They also used a mixture of Rooibos and mud which they applied to their heads and faces to ward off evil spirits.

In a study carried out by a French laboratory, Rooibos was found to positively affect the condition of hair and hair growth. When the results were tallied, respondents saw a reduction in hair loss, an improvement in the regrowth of hair and some even reported their hair had become smoother and more shiny.[35]

Beauty sleep

Sleep is the body's natural restoration period when it rejuvenates and repairs itself. Not getting enough sleep can release stress hormones into your system that cause your hair to stop growing or slow down your hair's natural growth cycle.

The Facts: Sleep is essential for the normal functioning of all systems in the body. Cells divide, tissue synthesises and growth hormones are released during sleep.

When our sleep suffers, our hair can too. Sleep deprivation is a form of stress that can trigger hair loss. When we do not get enough of our beauty sleep, our cortisol levels can increase. Elevated cortisol levels have been linked to inhibiting hair growth as they affect thyroid function.[36]

Adequate, uninterrupted sleep (6-8 hours) can significantly help alleviate cortisol levels and the associated anxiety, depression, stress or anger that comes from lack of sleep.

Bed head

Here's a secret hairdressers have know for decades (and the Chinese have known for centuries). Silk and satin pillowcases are gentler on your hair than cotton. Get yourself a silk pillowcase and say goodbye to the dreaded morning 'bird's nest' and 'hello' to sexy tousled morning hair.

The Facts: When you sleep on a silk or satin pillowcase, you will notice a huge amount of difference in the state of your hair when you wake up in the morning.

Silk allows your hair to glide over the pillow, rather than grabbing it every time you move your head during the night. Less friction means less tangling and pulling, which in turn means less hair loss.

Satin is a cheaper more durable alternative to silk if cost is an issue.

Cotton pillowcases have the tendency to dry out hair by drawing out moisture. The rough treatment on coarse cotton causes bed-head and can also damage your hair follicles, leading to thinner, less healthy hair.

The thief in the night

Each night you may be unknowingly robbing yourself of healthy hair. A pillow covered with hair each morning is usually a good indicator of the damage you are doing in your sleep.

The Facts: Even with the appropriate pillow case, your sleep style, especially if you are restless, can be causing damage to your hair

Night-time hair protection is important when you are trying to grow your hair and guard it against accidental breakage. Braiding or bunning your hair at night will protect it from friction, pulling and knots.

Application of oils or leave-in treatments will give additional protection and lessen knots and tangles from forming.

Pest protection

Pesky nits are an unwelcome pest guest for hair and they have a tendency to keep coming back. Any parent whose child has had them knows the embarrassment associated with being told their child "has nits". The persistent scratching can damage and irritate the scalp and lead to hair that is knotty and full of tangles, plus it is a dead giveaway that you (or your child) are the host carrying the infestation.

The Facts: Head lice can be eliminated without using toxic harsh chemicals and without spending lots of money. The key is in the comb. A recent study found that using a fine tooth comb especially designed for head lice on wet hair was four times more effective in getting rid of head lice than head lice shampoos.[37]

However, combing with such a fine utensil can be damaging to your fragile, wet hair. Coating the hair in coconut oil makes it easier for the comb to glide through the hair and has been found to be effective in the war against head lice by suffocating adult and juvenile nits.[38]

Many lice have become resistant to the most commonly used pesticides in lice shampoos. The health-conscious approach is one which does not seek to apply pesticides or insecticides to the scalp and have it absorbed into the blood to be circulated throughout the body.

According to researchers, neem seed oil is an effective natural head lice remedy and is highly effective against all stages of head lice.[38]

Coochie creme?

Miconazole nitrate, found in vaginal antifungal cremes, has been discussed for years in forums, chat rooms and medical sites as a way to accelerate hair growth. I kid you not!

The Facts: Miconazole nitrate is the active ingredient in antifungal creams such as Daktarin ® and Monistat ®. Normal use of these creams includes topical application for vaginal yeast infections, athlete's foot, ringworm and jock itch.

One theory is that miconazole nitrate aids in hair growth because it's an anti-fungal and this inhibits the growth of fungus on your scalp.

Another theory is that the nitrates widen and relax capillaries,[40] which improves circulation of oxygen to the hair. Blood circulation and oxygen levels directly stimulate the hair follicles, which leads to hair growth.

Whatever the explanation, it appears that, for some, increased hair growth is a positive side effect of this coochie cream.

Warning: Negative side effects that may arise from using miconazole nitrate for non-prescribed purposes can include headaches, hives and skin rashes.

Not your average garden variety herb

It seems the hippies and new-age gurus of yesteryear that reeked of patchouli oil were not just spouting nonsense when it came to the use of essential oils and their potential health benefits. In fact, aromatherapy oils have been anecdotally used to treat hair loss for hundreds of years.

The Facts: The natural essential oils from plant materials used for aromatherapy promote health and wellbeing. Essential oils are not actually oils, but have very similar characteristics, and are not to be confused with 'fragrant oils' which are synthetic substitutes used in many hair care products.

The 5,000-year-old science of extracting essential oils is one of the earliest forms of medicine. The resurgence of alternative medicine is a testament to the growing public interest in the health-promoting and medicinal properties of natural and organic resources.

A recent study showed active stimulants for hair growth are present in aromatherapy blends of essential oils.[41] The results of the study showed aromatherapy to be a safe and effective treatment, which had a positive effect on remedying alopecia areata for almost half the participants.

Rosemary (Rosmarinus officinalis):

Since the time of the ancient Egyptians, rosemary has been used to stimulate hair growth. It is one of the best herbs to use as a tonic and conditioner, as it gives lustre and body. Rosemary can also slightly darken the hair. It's full of micronutrients and antibacterial agents that are beneficial for the scalp.

Cedarwood extract (Cedrus atlantica/Juniperus virginiana):

Cedarwood extract is used in conjunction with scalp massages to assist oxygen getting into the hair follicle. This oil has a number of therapeutic benefits to assist hair growth: fungicide, antiseptic, astringent and antiseborrhoeic (relieves excess sebum secretion). In Europe, it is included in commercial shampoos and lotions for alopecia.

Lavender (Lavandula angustifolia/Lavandula officinalis):

Lavender has both antiseptic and antibiotic properties and assists in drawing blood to the scalp which helps prevent hair loss. Numerous studies have provided scientific evidence that aromatherapy with lavender oils also helps improve sleep and promote relaxation.[42]

Stinging nettle (Urtica dioica):

Stinging nettle has been used for years to prevent hair loss and to encourage hair growth.

Research has found that nettle root extract partially blocks the enzymes which are involved in the synthesis of dihydrotestosterone.[43] Too high levels of dihydrotestosterone (DHT) contribute to baldness (see *Hormone havoc* chapter).

The irritant effect of stinging nettle is thought to assist in hair growth by aiding circulation.

Saw palmetto (Serenoa repens):

Saw palmetto is another herb known to inhibit the enzyme DHT.[44] In some cases, it can stop or at least slow the rate of hair loss.

Catnip (Nepeta cataria):

Catnip is highly recommended to prevent split ends. The vitamin E oil found in catnip make it a fantastic conditioning treatment; it won't fix split ends but it can help make your hair stronger and prevent split ends from forming in the first place.

Riding the horsetails

It seems even the name of this tea, horsetail, conjures up images of a long, enviable mane of hair.

The Facts: Horsetail tea contains high concentrations of silicic acid, potassium and manganese. The high silica content supports the amino acids that build protein, resulting in hair that has better tensile strength and is less likely to fall out. Its high potassium content also makes it good for the heart and the circulatory system. A healthy circulatory system speeds nutrients from the blood to the scalp so that the hair is fed and grows.

Indian influence

After watching many Indian Bollywood movies, it is easy to come to the realisation that Indian women know a thing or two about hair care. Ayurvedic hair oils are known throughout India to effectively promote hair growth and have been touted as useful in the treatment of alopecia.

The Facts: Ayurveda (The Science of Life) is an ancient holistic medicine of India using particular herbs to heal and prolong life. Ayurvedic herbs used for hair care contribute to improving blood circulation, disinfecting the scalp and overall hair health. I have compiled a list of common herbs used in Indian haircare products.

Liquorice extract (Glycyrrhiza glabra, Glycyrrhiza uralensis):

Liquorice extract prevents hair fall and can suppress excessive scalp sebum secretion that can lead to scalp fungal infections. Liquorice affects all hormone secretions in the body, including oestrogen. Studies show that liquorice is antibacterial and anti-inflammatory, and affects oestrogenic activity.[45]

Fenugreek (Trigonella foenum-graecum):

A potent herb which has been found to increase hair growth, fenugreek contains vitamin B3, which assists in scalp circulation. The herb also contains a large amount of lecithin, a natural emollient known to strengthen dry, damaged hair, as well as biotin and inositol which are both known to spur on hair growth.

Packed with such powerful nutrients, fenugreek is used by many herbalists and beauticians to promote hair growth, lustre, health and shine.

Amla (Emblica officinalis):

One of the world's oldest natural hair conditioners, amla oil, derived from the amalaki fruit has been used in India for centuries. Known also as the Indian gooseberry, amla oil is packed with vitamin C, along with several other nutrients such as antioxidants, protein, calcium, iron, phosphorus and carotene.

Amla oil's astringent properties have been used as a conditioner to treat hair loss, premature greying, weakening of roots and dandruff. When mixed with a base oil, amla nourishes the hair to make it softer.

Taken internally, amla oil promotes hair health by correcting poor digestion which in turn affects the absorption of nutrients.

Brahmi (Bacopa monnieri):

As a nerve tonic herb, brahmi is known for its calming effects and anxiety reduction properties. It has antioxidant properties that allow nourishment to reach the hair roots and thus promote growth.

Brahmi is an essential component of many Indian herbal hair oils. Using this oil tends to cool the scalp and thus relax brain activity, inducing a good and restful sleep.[46]

Gotu Kola (Centella asiatica):

This herb promotes circulation and encourages the repair and regeneration of damaged tissue. One of its constituents, asiaticoside, works to stimulate skin repair and to strengthen skin, hair, nails and connective tissue.[47]

Bringraj (Eclipta alba, Eclipta prostrata):

Bhringraj, which literally translates to "king of hair", is used to regrow hair. Studies show the herb to be an effective treatment for alopecia.[48]

Bhringraj is a main ingredient in many ayurvedic herbal hair oils used for prevention of premature balding and promoting hair growth. The leaf extract is considered to be a powerful liver tonic and is also used for treating fungal infections.[49]

Hibiscus (Rosa sinensis):

Hibiscus acts as a natural emollient hair conditioner.[50] Used as a hair rinse, it stimulates thicker hair growth, and prevents greying, hair loss and scalp disorders. Its ingestion aids in the strengthening of hair roots whilst nourishing the hair from deep within.

One clinical study showed that the leaf extract of the hibiscus increased hair length and the anagen/telogen ratio of hair follicles.[51] The study concluded that the leaf extract, when compared to flower extract, exhibits a more potent effect on hair growth.

Glossy Privet (Lucidum ligustrum):

Used as a kidney and liver tonic, lucidum can improve circulation to the scalp, helping with hair restoration and preventing hair loss. Studies have shown lucidum ligustrum contains ursolic and oleanolic acid.[52] Oleanolic acid encourages hair growth by stimulating the peripheral blood flow in the scalp.

Shikakai/Sheekakai (Acacia concinna):

Traditionally used as a natural shampoo in India, shikakai has a naturally low pH. This makes for a very mild wash for your hair because it doesn't strip shafts of their natural oils. An infusion of the leaves can be used in anti-dandruff preparations.

Chinese whispers

In traditional China (and much of modern China), herbs are known to be of high value for medicines. Several of the traditional Indian Ayurverdic herbs, such liquorice extract, fenugreek and lucidum ligustrum, have also been used for centuries by the Chinese.

He shou wu, also known as the *fo ti* herb, is a Chinese secret to healthy hair. The Chinese say that long-term use of this famous 'longevity' herb helps return an aging person to youthfulness.

The Facts: *He Shou Wu (Polygonum multiflorum)*

The literal translation of *he shou wu* is "black-haired Mr. He". This refers to the Chinese legend where 'Mr. He' returned from living in the woods for some time and his grey hair had turned to black.

As it turned out, Mr. He had been consuming the *fo ti* herb to survive. *Fo ti* is known in China as the best herb to restore hair colour and nourish the skin, hair, teeth and nails. This popular Chinese herb is also used as a blood tonic for its cleansing effects.

Research of the plant's compounds has found *he shou wu* to be a natural anti-androgen, and a testosterone and DHT reductant (see *Hormone Havoc* chapter). It can stop hair loss by helping block the conversion of testosterone into follicle-shrinking DHT.[53]

Treatment with *he shou wu* can also help increase the blood supply within hair follicles, which can help optimise hair growth.[54]

It's all in your head

One of the things I miss most about visiting the hairdressing salon is the scalp massages. They not only feel so good, they are often overlooked as part of the healthy hair care regime. A relaxing scalp massage will stimulate your blood circulation,[55] release stress and nourish and strengthen your hair follicles.

The Facts: When there is an insufficient blood flow to the hair follicle, hair is more likely to go into the resting phase prematurely or become weak and brittle. Remember, if the hair goes into the resting phase, it is shed so that new hair can begin to take its place. But if hair prematurely enters the resting phase, there could be an abundance of hair being shed at one time, which will give the appearance of thinning hair.

A healthy scalp is essential for you to have a shiny, well-conditioned head of hair. More blood to the roots will help the hair follicles become nourished by nutrients and oxygen. Nourishment strengthens the roots of your hair, which leads to stronger hair that is less likely to break.

Your hair will be able to experience maximum health with regular scalp stimulation, and your follicles will be stimulated to produce more hair more quickly.

Indian hair bullying

An Indian parent at my daughter's school told me about hair pulling when we were discussing the disappointing state of my hair. As a practitioner of Auyverdic medicine he mentioned hair pulling to stimulate growth, which I will refer to as Indian hair pulling, not to be confused with trichotillomania or obsessive hair pulling.

The Facts: Indian hair pulling stimulates the circulation of the scalp by gently tugging wads of hair. It has a similar effect to scalp massage, by stimulating blood flow/circulation.

An interesting theory behind Indian hair pulling is that the arrector pili (the band of muscle tissue which connects the hair follicle to the scalp and is responsible for "lifting" the hair for goose bumps) is gently worked and strengthened.[11]

Turning heads

Shrinking capillaries or scalp muscle tension can cause a lack of blood flow to the scalp. Inversion is the simple method of inverting your body so more blood flows to your head. You can do this by letting half your body hang off the side of a bed, performing headstands or bending at the waist and flipping your hair over.

The Facts: Leaning forward helps the blood flow to the scalp and this helps strengthen the hair follicles.

Inversion needs to be practised somewhere safe so you do not end up head over tail in the bathroom recess from losing your balance and slipping on shampoo. There is also the swollen head effect, whereby you can actually feel your face filling up with blood and your eyes feel a little bulgy, do not stress this will pass, just don't hold the pose too long and practise your inversion in moderation.

Hormone havoc

During our teens, hormones like to play havoc on our skin whereas our hair seems to be resilient and immune to damage. Looking back to when I was a teenager, I remember having thick locks of hair which I loved to torture nearly every month with different colours and hairstyles. As we move from our teens to adulthood our hormone levels begin to change. The high levels of oestrogen we once had start to decline, male hormones may start to dominate and stress hormones begin to rise, our hair is no longer what it once used to be. As we age our hormones tend to start a different assault, this time on our hair.

The Facts: Our hair lives under hormonal dependence. The hormone oestrogen (estrogen) generally encourages hair to grow on the head. Testosterone, found in higher levels in males, governs body hair growth, such as a beard, underarm hair and pubic hair.

As women age and approach menopause, their bodies begin to produce less oestrogen, these lower levels of oestrogen can be associated with hair loss and thinning hair. Several studies have shown that oestrogen supplementation for women affected by hair loss leads to less shedding and an increase in hair thickness.[54] Higher testosterone levels can also make your hair thin and cause your head to produce less hair. Topical treatments with oestrogen have also been known to successfully restore hair growth and stop hair loss.[56]

During pregnancy, women produce higher concentrations of oestrogen which can result in the development of thicker, stronger, longer and healthier looking hair. The hair cycle tends to shed less and grow more during this period. Women are prone to temporary hair loss immediately after pregnancy because the extended hair growth stops and these hairs go into their 'resting phase' before embarking on their regular pre-pregnancy cycle.

Hormonal contraceptives can have a negative or a positive impact on the health of your hair. Depending on its composition, 'the pill' can amplify or even trigger hair problems, or fix these issues. Many androgenic oral contraceptives (containing testosterone and low doses of oestrogen) can decrease hair growth.

Androgenetic alopecia, otherwise know as male pattern hair loss, is believed to be due to the conversion of testosterone into dihydrotestosterone (DHT). Researchers nominate DHT as one of the primary contributors to male pattern hair loss,[54] which can occur in both men and women.

It's important to note that not all hormonal imbalances are related to testosterone and oestrogen levels. Some can be caused by a thyroid dysfunction, infection or an undiagnosed illness.

Pumpkin seeds – a special mention

I have repeatedly discovered during my hair research a link between prostate cancer studies and hair loss remedies. I was somewhat surprised when I stumbled upon research linking the humble pumpkin seed, otherwise known as pepitas, as a simple remedy for hair loss.

The Facts: Pumpkin seeds are a good source of protein and unsaturated fatty acids. They have long been an ancient Egyptian and Eastern European folk remedy for men's health issues.[57]

Many health professionals claim that pumpkin seeds are effective against hair loss. A recent study found that pumpkin seeds lower testosterone levels, which can be helpful in reducing hair loss.[57]

The humble pumpkin seed affects the levels of androgen production and inhibits DHT.[44] Androgen is the male hormone that plays a very important role in hair loss and hair growth. Increases in DHT can be responsible for shrinking the hair follicle. When the hair follicle gets smaller and finer, the hair then falls out. DHT also creates a wax-like substance around the hair roots and it is this accumulation of DHT in the hair follicles and roots that can give rise to male and female pattern hair loss.[58]

Don't stress me out

A too stressful lifestyle can alter the growth cycle of your hair and can prematurely terminate the normal duration of active hair growth.

The Facts: Stress is a natural part of life. Too much prolonged stress, however, can accelerate and aggravate hair loss by increasing your testosterone levels and put hair into a dormant resting phase.[59]

A condition called stress alopecia results when a large number of hair follicles prematurely enter the resting phase and fall out at the same time.[60] Stress alopecia can occur with:

- Certain medications
- Nutritional deficiencies
- Surgery
- Illness

- Exams

- Divorce

- Child birth

- Sleep deprivation

- Dehydration

- Life's trivialities

Basically, any chronic stressful life experiences can affect your hair's health.

The impact on your hair from a stressful event can sometimes occur 3-4 months after the event has passed. The ability to relax and let go of worries will determine your stress levels.

Lifestyle

At the risk of sounding like the proverbial broken record, lifestyle affects every part of your life, even your hair's growth and health.

The Facts: Put simply, exercise increases blood circulation, whereas alcohol depletes your body of essential nutrients and smoking cigarettes reduces blood flow.

Each of these factors has a significant influence on the health of your scalp, and an unhealthy scalp will cause a reduction in hair growth.

A watched pot never boils

Growing hair long and healthy will take commitment, and you will have to make sacrifices. This may mean giving up your favourite styling technique and other lifestyle changes.

The Facts: Your hair can grow from between a few millimetres to a couple of centimetres every month. Genetics and diet play a major role in your hair's ability to grow. The amount of hair that breaks off or you cut off will also affect the time it takes to grow your hair too.

Growing out damage will take time; during that time you can be proactive in taking good care of your hair to stop further damage and to support new growth.

Lifestyle changes will take around three months to result in real hair improvements, so patience is essential.

Author's note: Hair is only hair

Hair is only hair and for most of us it will grow back even after we continue to damage and torture it.

For some of us our hair defines us and it can be emotionally devastating when our hair falls out or just looks and feels wrong. If you are at your wits end and threatening to shave it off and start again, please try some or all of the tips and ideas listed in the **Appendices** before doing anything too drastic.

In conclusion, to achieve the longest, healthiest hair possible, you need to consider doing the following:

Stop hair breakage/damage before it happens

Minimising hair breakage will allow your hair to reach its maximum length. Protect your hair using specific types of products (as suggested in this book), as part of a hair care regime which can help reduce breakage and increase your hair length.

Increase the growth phase and lessen shedding

Using hair vitamins and mineral supplements to complement a healthy eating plan will naturally lengthen your hair's anagen phase and allow your hair to grow much longer before it enters the resting and shedding phases. Get plenty of rest and practise positive stress management.

Improve the health of your hair before it starts to grow

A healthy, bacteria-free, well-nourished scalp enables you to grow lush, long, healthy hair.

Appendix I

Over 50 Tips & Ideas to longer, healthier hair

Tips and Ideas

Tip 1: Coconut oil can be used as the perfect daily moisturiser. Simply put a small amount in the palms of your hands, rub together and apply to hair strands to keep hair moisturised.

Tip 2: Experiment with different oils like olive, mineral, avocado, almond and jojoba to trial which ones are right for you and work best with your hair type.

Tip 3: Castor Oil has been used for centuries in India to assist hair growth and to thicken hair.

Idea 1: Castor oil growth recipe

Castor oil is quite thick and sticky so it needs to be blended with other oils to ensure it does not accidentally rip your hairs out whilst you massage with it.

1.Mix 50mls of Castor oil with 50mls of your favourite carrier oil (Coconut, Avocado, Almond, Jojoba or Olive oil).

2.Apply to your hair roots, massage into scalp and then leave on overnight (or for at least half an hour).

3.Shampoo hair to remove Castor Oil residue

4.For maximum effect use three times a week

Tip 4: Argan oil locks in moisture and cures hair of brittleness.

Tip 5: Any process which uses chemicals to alter the structure of the hair will compromise the internal structure of your hair, weakening it and making it more susceptible to further damage. Over time and with repeated use it will leave your hair dry, dull, weak or frizzy and at greater risk of damage from the daily hair care routine.

Tip 6: Using henna helps smooth the cuticle and your hair is naturally plumped with volume from within, taking on a thicker, stronger texture. Henna stains hair to the desired colour without chemically damaging the hair structure. It can leave hair feeling gritty so use a deep conditioning agent for a couple of days after application.

Idea 2: Changing the shades of Henna

Red Henna (Lawsonia inermis): Provides a red stain, deepen by mixing and letting sit overnight in an iron pot, or accent with burgundy streaks by adding raw beetroot juice. Copper piping or pennies will add brown hues to red Henna. Adding natural yoghurt to your henna mix will help make application easier and give you a creamier consistency.

Black Henna (Indigofera tinctoria): Gives a deep black colouring.

Hendigo: A mix of henna and indigo in varying quantities will give different shades of browns including chestnut and mahogany.

Neutral Henna (Cassia obovata): has a golden dye molecule that will stain dull blonde and gray hair yellow. Cassia treatments can be used on dark tresses for shine enhancement.

Tip 7: Bleaching the hair is a very harsh process and should be avoided. It compromises the internal hair structure and can have devastating results if you aren't careful. The lighter you take your hair from its natural colour, the more damage will occur. Natural alternatives to chemical bleaching include Cinnamon essential oil, Baking Soda, Honey, Sunshine and Lemon Citrus essential oil.

Idea 3 Coconut oil presoak

Presoaking your hair with coconut oil will help your hair survive the damage harsh bleach can have on your hair. Ultimately you will have less of the damage usually associated with having hair chemically lightened.

1.Two days before having your hair bleached or highlighted, oil your hair with coconut oil.

2.Apply a liberal amount of virgin coconut oil to your entire hair shaft, root to tip. Leave in and do not wash out.

3.There's no need to wash it out each night or morning until the day you are due to start the bleaching

4.It is optional whether or not to remove the oil before bleaching agents are applied to your hair. The oil should not effect the strength of the chemicals.

Tip 8: Regardless of whether you visit a hair salon or colour, bleach or perm your hair at home, chemical processing damages your hair.

Tip 9: Excessive friction from manual hairstyling, like over-zealous brushing, backcombing or teasing, can damage and affect the health of your hair. If you choose to brush your hair, do it gently. To test if your brush or technique is costing you precious hairs, brush dry hair over a white sink and check for breakage. For people with thinning hair, every hair counts, harsh brushing can often pull out hair that would not have come out had you not brushed it.

Tip 10: Raking the wrong type of brush through your hair and brushing when wet makes your hair highly vulnerable to damage. The best way to detangle hair following a wash is by using a wide-toothed comb. Try to avoid using a hair brush until your hair is almost dry. If you must brush, lubricate your hair first with your favourite oils.

Tip 11: Using your hands and a small amount of your favourite oil or conditioner to gently untangle knots is a lot gentler and less aggressive way to avoid pulling hairs out by the roots or snapping hair. Fingercombing in the shower will also enhance curls.

Tip 12: Feel a comb or brush bristles for any rough or sharp areas before you purchase it. Sharp seams and plastic nibs catch on delicate long hair and promote breakage. Buy handmade wood or seamless plastic combs which will glide through your hair without catching on fragile strands. A good way to check if your current comb or brush is damaging your hair is to stand over a white sink whilst you groom your hair, if there is a large number of hairs breaking off you'll see them.

Tip 13: Hair is like string and will start to unravel regardless of where you cut it. Try 1/2 cm trims (only when you need to) to maintain healthy ends. Clean ends tangle less and will break less. Your faster growing hairs will be trimmed back regularly so that slower growing hairs can 'catch up', giving you less wispy ends and a thicker hemline.

Tip 14: Find a hairdresser that knows how to micro-trim. Speak up when in the hairdresser's chair, your hairdresser will appreciate your input and you are less likely to leave with your hair butchered into a style you really did not want.

Tip 15: Use warm water to wash or clarify, this opens up your hair cuticles and helps your conditioner or herbal rinse to penetrate the hair. Use cool water on low pressure to rinse and to close the cuticle. Alternating between hot and cold whilst in the shower also improves circulation to the scalp.

Tip 16: Keep your body and hair hydrated by drinking plenty of fresh clean water. Monitor your water intake.

Tip 17: There are several water contaminants that can cause hair loss, if these contaminants are in your water, try using a filtered showerhead.

Tip 18: Protect hair with a swim cap when swimming in chlorine or saltwater, saturate with water and oil before getting in the water and rinse with club soda afterwards. Wetting the hair with non-chlorinated water prior to swimming in pools and the ocean will lessen the amount of chlorine and salt water elements absorbed into the hair shaft.

Idea 4: Baking Soda Shampoo Recipe

An effective alternative to using Chelating shampoos to remove chlorine and mineral deposits from your hair

1.Mix 1/2 teaspoon baking soda in 1litre of water and pour onto your scalp

2.Gently massage baking soda rinse into your hair

3.Rinse hair with warm water

4.Condition hair and rinse again with Apple Cider Vinegar rinse.

Tip 19: Although not the most attractive accessory, swimming caps are well-suited for protecting hair. For those with long hair, caps can also help hair from dragging along during laps becoming prone to more tangles.

Tip 20: Some of us have hair that can be damaged by chemicals in shampoos. Alternatives to using your current shampoo regime are worth considering; you just need to find what works for you.

Idea 5: Shampooing Alternatives

•Shampoo bars or baby shampoos which are ph balanced.

•Organic shampoos, but check the ingredients first for hidden nasties.

•Baking Soda in place of shampoo will cleanse the hair just as effectively without stripping it of moisture, but may lighten hair.

•Pre-oiling the scalp and hair with your favorite oils prior to washing to prevent the protein loss in response to shampooing

•Adding Coconut oil to shampoo to lessen the harshness of your current shampoo.

•Experiment with conditioning your hair first then washing followed by more conditioner

•Only wash with a conditioner

•Shampooing less frequently may help avoiding drying hair out.

Tip 21: You can still have your crowning glory shine and glow without the use of alcohol based styling products. There are many natural alcohol-free gels and sprays out there. A light oiling with Argan or your favourite oil can keep hair from being flyaway. On its own or diluted with water into a spray bottle Aloe Vera works wonders as a natural styling agent.

Tip 22: Naturally healthy hair needs a natural approach. Look for cone free and sulfate free shampoos and conditioners that do not contain harsh chemicals. Alternatively, go natural and use an apple cider vinegar rinse to remove build up, baking soda shampoos and oils for frizz free hair and leave in conditioning.

Tip 23: Protein treatments put protein back into your hair but should always be followed with a deep conditioning treatment. Homemade Egg, Soy Sauce or Gelatin protein treatments will save you money and still give good results

Idea 6: Raw Egg Protein Treatment Recipe

Recommended once a month if your hair is not dry and brittle.

1.Separate the yolk from the whites of two eggs and beat.

Only use the yolk of the egg for your protein masque, the whites will cause excessive dryness.

2.Apply the yolk mixture to dry hair and leave on for 30mins

3.Gently rinse hair with warm water.

4.Always follow your protein treatment with a deep conditioning treatment

Tip 24: Unrefined Shea Butter is full of vitamins and is a natural moisturiser. Its emollient properties relieve scalp dryness and leaves hair feeling silky and soft.

Idea 7: Deep Conditioning Recipe

Shea Butter deep conditioning masque

Recommended once a fortnight if your hair is dry and brittle.

1.Blend 2 tablespoons of Shea Butter with 1 tbls Coconut oil, Avocado or Olive Oil and 1 tbls of your favourite All Natural conditioner.

2.Apply to damp hair and leave on for 1-4hrs.

3.Rinse hair. Shampoo and condition

Tip 25: Apple Cider Vinegar is an excellent clarifying rinse to remove build up and cleanse your scalp.

Idea 8: ACV Rinse Recipe

Use once a week after washing to clarify and remove build up

1.Combine one to two tablespoons of ACV with one cup of water.

2.After washing pour the rinse over your hair

3.Do not rinse out, the vinegar 'smell' will abate once your hair has dried

Caution: Never mix Apple Cider Vinegar with Baking powder you could 'melt' your hair!

Tip 26: Torturing hair into submission damages your hair and causes breakage. Trying to attain a style that may not suit you is time consuming, expensive and could be costing you precious hairs. It may be time to stop fighting genetics and accept your hair type. Embrace your curls, kinks or individual style.

Tip 27: Chemical relaxing or straightening is never to the benefit to your hair's health. Regardless of which method of straightening you use, this type of hairstyling is extremely damaging.

Tip 28: Using heat to style hair can cause damage and dry out hair. Use the cooler settings on your hairdryer or avoid heat styling altogether.

Tip 29: Showers that are too hot can damage your hair, keep showers and bath water warm, not hot.

Tip 30: Heat can aid deep conditioners to penetrate the hair shaft by opening the cuticle, being especially beneficial for conditioning treatments on dry hair.

Idea 9: Coconut Oil Heat Treatment

1.Apply warm Coconut Oil to scalp and damp hair

2.Heat a towel in the microwave for 1minute or until warm

3.Wrap hair in warm towel

The hot towel will open the cuticles and allow the Coconut Oil to penetrate deep inside the hair shaft

4.Leave on for 30mins then rinse, wash out or use as leave in conditioner

Tip 31: Sock buns give curls and volume to straight or limp hair without the use of damaging heat.

Idea 10: How to make Sock Bun

1.Cut the foot off a long sock and roll it into a donut shape.

2.Comb your hair into a not-too-tight ponytail on top of your head (either use a band you do not mind snipping off or wrap a finger-width strand of hair around your tail and pin into place).

3.Lightly moisturise the ponytail using your favourite oil

4.Put the end of your ponytail into the donut opening.

5.Tuck the end of your tail up into the outside of the sock donut.

6.Now roll the donut down your ponytail until it's flush against your scalp.

Try and spread the hair evenly over the donut ensuring it doesn't show through

7.You may want to secure the sock in place with a bobby pin.

8.Leave in for a couple of hours or overnight to set.

9.Remove the sock and reveal your luscious lovely sock-bun curls

Tip 32: A Doobie will protect your hair while you sleep, exercise or even whilst doing your chores! When you take the Doobie out you'll notice your hair feels smooth, straight and tangle-free.

Idea 11: How to Doobie Your Hair

1.Start with clean, air dried and combed hair.

2.Be sure to comb your hair all in the same direction (i.e., to one side)

3.Take the ends of your hair and 'wrap' around your head, as far as you can

(Longer hair may wrap around all the way or more than once).

4.Secure your hair with bobby pins to keep it in place.

5.Protect with a headband or bandanna.

Tip 33: Switch up your hair part lines alternating from side parts and centre parts. Find your new part and pin it down with bobby pins as soon as you get out of the shower (so that it dries parted to the side). This technique trains your hair to lay which ever way you want it to.

Tip 34: Loose braids and bunning your hair without the use of over tight elastic bands will save your hair from accidental breakage during the day. Mix up styles to avoid Hair Repetitive Stress Injuries (RSI), even placing your ponytail in different locations (high, low and to the side) helps.

Tip 35: Seek the expertise of your Health Practitioner to determine any vitamin and mineral deficiencies. In combination with a healthy eating plan it is critical you are getting the correct doses of the vitamins and minerals you need. Pregnant and

Breastfeeding mums and children will require different recommended daily amounts.

Tip 36: Studies show a direct correlation to hair loss and vitamin D deficiency. Spending a few minutes in the Sun is enough to get your daily dose. Wear a hat to protect your hair (and face) from Sun exposure.

Tip 37: The nutritional benefits of nuts can't be overlooked, eat a variety of nuts for best hair growth. The fats they contain are healthy fats and they make a great snack idea.

Tip 38: Diet and hair are linked. Follow the healthy hair diet if you want healthy beautiful hair eat healthy foods, avoid crash diets, and eat adequate amounts of protein, carbohydrates, fruit and vegetables, low-fat dairy and 'good' fats for your body type or lifestyle. A dietician or your Health Provider can assist you in creating a hair healthy eating plan suitable to your individual needs.

Idea 12: Conditioning Banana Hair Masque Recipe

1.Freeze a banana; this makes it easier to mush.

2.Use a blender or food processor to puree the banana until it is liquefied (Make sure it's totally smooth otherwise you'll end up with banana chunks stuck in your hair).

3.Blend the banana with a mashed avocado and a teaspoon of Olive oil or Coconut Oil.

(Avocados are packed with fatty acids that will soften the hair)

4.Once blended, scoop the mixture on to your damp hair.

5.Cover with a shower cap or plastic wrap and relax for 15 minutes.

6.Rinse with cool water.

Tip 39: For the internal benefits of Molasses take 1 tablespoon of blackstrap molasses first thing in the morning. Be careful, some people find molasses can have a laxative effect.

Idea 13: Topically applied Molasses hair rinse

1.Add one tablespoon of molasses to a cup of warm water

2.Massage mixture into the hair.

(Make sure to completely cover the roots to stimulate hair growth)

3.After half an hour, rinse off with warm water. Then shampoo and condition as usual.

Tip 40: Rooibos tea has independent lab data to show it improves hair growth and condition hair. Brew and steep your Rooibos tea until cooled, then pour over hair as a hair rinse. Rinsing with Rooibos after showering also helps lessen frizz.

Tip 41: Make time to sleep and get enough shut-eye every night. You can indulge your strands whilst you sleep with a night time masque or leave-in conditioner.

Tip 42: Oil and loose braid your hair before going to bed to limit damage from when you are asleep. Silk pillowcases cause less friction when you move around at night and can help to prevent split ends whilst locking in your hair's natural oils.

Tip 43: If you want your hair to grow it is very important for you to manage your stress in positive ways. This means taking care of your health through diet and exercise and finding ways to relieve and avoid stress.

Tip 44: Wear your hair up so as to avoid hair snagging and to protect it from the elements. Be inventive and find new and exciting ways to wear your hair. Try to wear your hair out on special occasions only.

Tip 45: Chemicals from lice treatments can dry out hair and are absorbed into the blood stream. If you decide to continue using over the counter medicated headlice treatments, apply coconut or olive oil to your ends so they don't dry out.

Idea 14: Natural Nit Treatment Recipe

1.Add 20 - 30 ml of Neem oil to your shampoo

2.Leave in your hair for 10 minutes.

3.Rinse well and condition, before rinsing again.

Regular washing with Neem shampoo will help you get rid of nits for good.

Tip 46: Fine tooth combs for lice removal can damage your hair, therefore apply a generous amount of coconut oil to your hair to assist the comb in gliding through your hair and to suffocate nits.

Tip 47: Antifungal cremes that contain Miconazole Nitrate can reduce the growth of scalp fungus and improve circulation to the scalp. Applying these cremes to the roots of your hair 2-3times a week can improve the growth rate of your hair.

Warning: Pregnant and Breastfeeding mothers should see their health provider before use.

Tip 48: Herbs can be taken orally or used as a rinse to stimulate the scalp and hair follicles. Finding the right herbal mix can effectively condition and strengthen your hair. You can boil them into a tea and infuse them into an after showering hair rinse. Otherwise use a little essential oil mixed with your favourite oil and massage into the scalp.

Tip 49: Horsetail can be brewed into a tea and taken internally or applied as an after shower hair rinse. Its high silica content helps build protein, making hair stronger.

Tip 50: Traditional medicines have been used for hundreds of years to treat dandruff, increasing blood circulation, scalp cleansing and reducing inflammation. A combination of one or more Ayurvedic and Chinese Herbs may just be the missing link in helping you achieve longer healthier hair.

Tip 51: Scalp massages stimulate circulation to nourish hair follicles. After showering, massage the scalp vigorously with your favourite oil until it starts to feel warm or for at least 5minutes every day.

Idea 15: Controlled Pulling 'How to'

Controlled Pulling should never hurt or uproot any hairs, if it does you are pulling too hard

1.Start by placing your fingers on the scalp and moving the scalp back and forth like you are adjusting a wig

2.Grasp random chunks of hair firmly by the roots and tug gently

(Avoid asking another person to help you with this, as they are 99.5% likely to get carried away doing it at your expense!)

3.Continue this routine until you have "pulled" the hair all over your scalp.

Tip 52: Inverting your head helps get circulation to your scalp. You can try inversion whilst you massage with your favourite oils, when washing your roots and when combing your hair.

Idea 16: Inversion Idea 'How to'

How to Invert your hair whilst standing

1.Bend at the waist

2.Hang your head forward and tuck your chin under so it touches your chest

3.Allow your hair to fall over the head so it hangs freely

Tip 53: See your Health practitioner and have your hormone levels checked. Also, if applicable, check the hormone levels on any birth control you may be taking.

Tip 54: It will take around three months for you to see changes in your hair when you adopt some of or all of these Tips and Ideas. Patience is key to growing longer hair.

Appendix II (Cheat sheet)

Stuff you can try, buy, do and avoid

Stuff you can buy and try

Coconut oil

Oils – jojoba, avocado, mineral, almond & olive oil

Argan oil

Castor Oil

Henna – indigo, hendigo, cassia

Natural hair lighteners - cinnamon, honey or lemon

Miconazole nitrate crème

Coconut oil shampoo

Baking soda shampoo

Wide tooth wood comb

Silk or satin pillowcase

Apple cider vinegar rinses

Molasses hair masque

Banana hair masque

Showerhead filter

Swim cap

Soda water rinses

Trial shampooing variations

Deep conditioning shea butter hair masque

Rooibos tea rinses

Neem lice treatments

Aromatherapy essential oils

Ayurvedic herbal teas & rinses

Chinese medicine

Stuff you can eat and drink

Healthy food

Vitamin & mineral supplements

Apple cider vinegar

Clean water

Rooibos tea

Horsetail tea

Nuts

Bananas

Pumpkin seeds

Increase protein intake

Iron rich food

Ayurvedic herbs

Stuff you can do NOW

Scalp massages

Microtrims

Cold water rinses

Braiding hair at night

Wear loose hairstyles

Wearing hair up during the day

Gentle brushing

Don't fight genetics, embrace your curls and kinks

Sunshine

Inversion

Patience

Sock buns

Hair wrapping

Indian hair pulling

Beauty sleep

Protect ends during nit treatments

Lifestyle changes

Hormones checked

Protein treatments

Finger combing

Natural styling products

Varying the position of hair parting

Blood tests for nutritional deficiencies

Speak up when in the hairdresser's chair

Stuff you can avoid doing

Chemical hair dyes

Chemical hair treatments – perms & straightening

Using excessive heat - blow driers, straighteners, curling wands & scalding hot showers

Over zealous dry brushing/wet brushing

Avoiding stress

Excessive hair cuts

Rough use of plastic brushes and combs

Bleaching

Salt water, treated water and hard water

Too much Sun exposure

Alcohol based synthetic styling products

Repetitive hairstyling

Backcombing & hair teasing

Harsh shampoos

Overtight braids and ponytails

Yoyo and Crash dieting

References

1. Ruetsch, S. B., Kamath, Y. K., Rele, A. S., & Mohile, R. B. (2001). Secondary ion mass spectrometric investigation of penetration of coconut and mineral oils into human hair fibers: Relevance to hair damage. Journal of Cosmetic Science, 52(3), 169-184.

2. Rele, A. S., & Mohile, R. B. (2002). Effect of mineral oil, sunflower oil, and coconut oil on prevention of hair damage. Journal of Cosmetic Science 54(2), 175-192.

3. Guillaume, D., & Charrouf, Z. (2011). Argan oil. Alternative Medicine Review, 16(3), 275-279.

4. Monfalouti, H. E., Guillaume, D., Denhez, C., & Charrouf, Z. (2010). Therapeutic potential of argan oil – A review. Journal of Pharmacy and Pharmacology, 62(12), 1669-1675

5. American Hair Loss Association. (2004-2010). Infectious Agents, from http://www.americanhairloss.org/types_of_hair_loss/infectious _agents.asp

6. Sukhvinder, S., Sandhu, S., & Robbins, C. R. (1993). A simple and sensitive technique, based on protein loss measurements, to assess surface damage to human hair. Journal of the Society of Cosmetic Chemists, 44, 163-175.

7. Jones, M. (2003). Healthy Hair with Henna, from http://www.byregion.net/articles-healers/Henna.html

8. Cartwright-Jones, C. (2005). The Enclyclopedia of Henna, from http://www.hennapage.com/henna/encyclopedia/

9. Fenton, C. (2011). Getting it straight: Untangling the Keratin Controversy, from http://stuffboston.com/stuffboston/archive/2011/05/02/getting-it-straight-untangling-the-keratin-controversy.aspx

10. Goldwert, L. (2011, April 14). Brazilian hair straightening hazardous: OSHA; Formaldehyde-free products found to contain carcinogen, Daily News. Retrieved from http://articles.nydailynews.com/2011-04-14/entertainment/29445369_1_formaldehyde-free-osha-products

11. Michael, G. (1981). Secrets for Beautiful Hair. Garden City, NY: Doubleday.

12. Gray, J. (2007). The World of Hair: Proctor & Gamble.

13. Watrous, L. M. (1997). Constitutional hydrotherapy: From nature cure to advanced naturopathic medicine. Journal of Naturopathic Medicine, 7(2), 72-79.

14. Dow Corporation. (2006). Product Safety, from http://www.dow.com/productsafety/finder/edta.htm

15. Terhanian, H. (1999). Warning: What Your Shampoo's Label Won't Tell You... from http://aztec.asu.edu/makingscents/articles/Shampoo/shampoo.html

16. Bouillon, C., & Wilkinson, J. (2005). The Science of Hair Care (2nd ed.): Taylor & Francis.

17. Maranz, S., Wiseman, Z., Bisgaard, J., & Bianchi, G. (2004). Germplasm resources of Vitellaria paradoxa based on variations in fat composition across the species distribution range.

Agroforestry Systems (in cooperation with ICRAF), 60(71). doi: 10.1023/B:AGFO.0000009406.19593.90.

18. Hardy, L. (2011, April 7). The hair-raising truth about straighteners: A third of women use them, but experts say hair irons can make your hair go more frizzy... and even fall out, Mail Online. Retrieved from http://www.dailymail.co.uk/femail/article-1364670/The-hair-raising-truth-straighteners-They-make-hair-fall-out.html

19. Dow Corning. (n.d.). Heat Protection for Hair Care, from http://www.dowcorning.com/content/publishedlit/HEATPRO TECT.pdf

20. BASF: The Chemical Company. (2007). Panthenol, from https://docs.google.com/viewer?a=v&q=cache:MfwkGpDaun EJ:www.basf.co.kr/02_products/04_finechemicals/cosmetics/d ata/Panthenol_MEMC060801e-01_Oct2007.pdf+topically+applied+Panthenol+study&hl=en& gl=au&pid=bl&srcid=ADGEEShXD3KrIF8KqcNbqLJuRFIG qeYl_oiusygUDC_igdXfTw0kNiGY_gKiVdQ2gu_zISTC4isfe6y 3ZUqgeyg_-PwE4ZHl8gx5pAbVx8ON2r5NSbE0cLjuQte3730lVZpTEdZh ATt5&sig=AHIEtbSUBRxN84f_ukMwxCNYFDQk9vC0sQ

21. Mayo Clinic. (2011). Folate, from http://www.mayoclinic.com/health/folate/NS_patient-folate/DSECTION=evidence%20THIS%20EVIDENCE-BASED%20MONOGRAPH%20WAS%20PREPARED%20B Y%20THE%20NATURAL%20STANDARD%20RESEARCH %20COLLABORATION%20(www.naturalstandard.com)%202 011

22. Linus Pauling Institute. (2000-2012). Biotin. Micronutrient Information Center, from http://lpi.oregonstate.edu/infocenter/vitamins/biotin/

23. Zhang, Y., Ni, J., Messing, E. M., Chang, E., Yang, C.-R., & Yeh, S. (2002). Vitamin E succinate inhibits the function of androgen receptor and the expression of prostate-specific antigen in prostate cancer cells. Proceedings of the National Academy of Sciences of the United States of America, 99(11), 7408-7413. doi: 10.1073/pnas.102014399.

24. Panin, G., Strumia, R., & Ursini, F. (2004). Topical alpha-tocopherol acetate in the bulk phase: Eight years of experience in skin treatment. Annals Of The New York Academy Of Sciences (2004), 1032, 443-447.

25. Cancer Council NSW. (2012). Vitamin D and sun protection, from http://www.cancercouncil.com.au/1815/reduce-risks/sun-protection/tips-for-being-be-sunsmart/tips-for-sun-protection/be-sunsmart/?pp=1815

26. Johnston, F. A., Debrock, L., & Diao, E. K. (1958). The loss of calcium, phosphorus, iron, and nitrogen in hair from the scalp of women. The American Journal of Clinical Nutrition, 6, 136-141.

27. Rushton, D. H. (2002). Nutritional factors and hair loss. Clinical and Experimental Dermatology, 27(5), 396-404.

28. Neve, H. J., Bhatti, W. A., Soulsby, C., Kincey, J., & Taylor, T. V. (1996). Reversal of hair loss following vertical gastroplasty when treated with zinc sulphate. Obes Surg, 6(1), 63-65

29. Cranton, E. M., & Passwater, R. A. (1983). Trace Elements, Hair Analysis and Nutrition: Keats Pub.

30. Lawrence, R. (2004). Essential Foods; Clinical Trial Report: The Effectiveness of the Use of Oral Lignisul MSM (Methylsulfonylmethane) Supplementation on Hair and Nail Health. Retrieved from http://www.essential-foods.co.uk/MSM-Studien/Lawrence-Hair-Nail-Report.htm

31. Ministry of Health. (n.d.). Protein. Nutrient Reference Values for Australia and New Zealand, from http://www.nrv.gov.au/nutrients/protein.htm

32. Bragg, P. C., & Bragg, P. (n.d.). Apple Cider Vinegar: Miracle Health System Retrieved from http://www.scribd.com/doc/47366689/Paul-C-Bragg-Apple-Cider-Vinegar-Miracle-Health-System

33. Buhl, A. E., Waldron, D. J., Conrad, S. J., Mulholland, S. J., Shull, K. L., Kubicek, M. F., Stehle, R. J. (1992). Potassium channel conductance: a mechanism affecting hair growth both in vitro and in vivo. The Journal of Investigative Dermatology, 98(3), 315-319.

34. Dr Oz Show. (Feb 28th 2010). USA.

35. Tiedtke, J., & Marks, O. (2011) Rooibos- the new "white tea" for hair and skin care retrieved from www.docstoc.com/docs/72640452/ROOIBOS---THE-NEW-%E2%80%9CWHITE-TEA%E2%80%9D-FOR-HAIR-AND-SKIN-CARE

36. Houssay, A. B., Epper, C. E., Varela, V., & Curbelo, H. M. (1978). Effects of halogenated analogues of cortisol and progesterone upon hair growth in castrated mice. Acta Physiol Lat Am, 28(1), 11-18.

37. Hill, N., Moor, G., Cameron, M. M., Butlin, A., Preston, S., Williamson, M. S., & Bass, C. (2005). Single blind, randomised, comparative study of the Bug Buster kit and over the counter

pediculicide treatments against head lice in the United Kingdom. British Medical Journal, 2005, 331-384.

38. Stuttaford, T. (2005) Lice: A natural solution at last The Times Newspaper (2005, July 8).

39. Abdel-Ghaffar, F., & Semmler, M. (2007). Efficacy of neem seed extract shampoo on head lice of naturally infected humans in Egypt. Parasitology Research, 100(2), 329-332.

40. Texas Heart Institute at St Luke's Episcopal Hospital. (2011). Nitrates,   from http://www.texasheart.org/HIC/Topics/Meds/nitrmeds.cfm

41. Hay, I. C., Jamieson, M., & Ormerod, A. D. (1998). Randomized trial of aromatherapy. Successful treatment for alopecia areata. Archives of Dermatology, 134(11), 1349-1352.

42. Lee, I. S., & Lee, G. J. (2006). Effects of lavender aromatherapy on insomnia and depression in women college students. Taehan Kanho Hakhoe Chi., 36(1), 136-143.

43. Hartmann, R. W., Mark, M., & Soldati, F. (1996). Inhibition of 5 alpha-reductase and aromatase by PHL-00801 (Prostatonin®), a combination of PY 102 (Pygeum africanum) and UR 102 (Uritca dioica) extracts. Phytomedicine, 3(2), 121-128.

44. Vahlensieck, W. (2002). With alpha blockers, finasteride and nettle root against benign prostatic hyperplasia. Which patients are helped by conservative therapy? MMW Fortschr Med., 144(16), 33-36.

45. Memorial Sloan-Kettering Cancer Center. (n.d.). Information About Herbs, Botanicals and Other Products, from http://www.mskcc.org/cancer-care/herb/licorice

46. Trivedi, H. (n. d.). Brahmi - Herbal Brain Tonic to Increase Memory:a review, from http://transradialformulations.academia.edu/HarshvardhanTrivedi/Papers/758786/Brahmi_-_Herbal_Brain_Tonic_to_Increase_Memory_a_review

47. MDidea Extracts Professional. (2010). Gotu Kola Centella asiatica, the Goddess of Supreme Wisdom, from http://www.mdidea.com/products/herbextract/gotukola/data06.html

48. Roy, R. K., Thakur, M., & Dixit, V. K. (2008). Hair growth promoting activity of Eclipta alba in male albino rats. Archives of dermatological research, 300(7), 357-364.

49. Dweck, A. C. (1975). Article for Cosmetics & Toiletries:Indian Plants. Retrieved from www.dweckdata.com/Published_papers/Indians.pdf

50. Gaur, K., Kori, M. L., & Nema, R. K. (2009). Comparative Screening of Immunomodulatory Activity of Hydro-alcoholic Extract of Hibiscus rosa sinensis Linn. and Ethanolic Extract of Cleome gynandr D Guillaume, H Monfalouti, C Denhez, Z Charrouf, 2010a Linn. Global Journal of Pharmacology, 3(2), 85-89.

51. Adhirajan, N., Ravi Kumar, T., Shanmugasundaram, N., & Babu, M. (2003). In vivo and in vitro evaluation of hair growth potential of Hibiscus rosa-sinensis Linn. Journal of Ethnopharmacology, 88(2-3), 235-239.

52. Xia, E.-Q., Wang, B.-W., Xu, X.-R., Zhu, L., Song, Y., & Li, H.-B. (2011). Microwave-Assisted Extraction of Oleanolic Acid and Ursolic Acid from Ligustrum lucidum Ait. International Journal

of Molecular Sciences, 12(8), 5319-5329. doi: http://dx.doi.org/10.3390/ijms12085319

53. American Botanical Council. (1999). Issue 46 HerbalGram. Spring 1999, from http://cms.herbalgram.org/herbalgram/issue.html?Issue=46

54. Kelley, C. (2006). Current State of Science Review focusing on characterization, efficacy and safety of Polygon(i)um Multiflorum Thunb for healthy hair. Herbal Hair Nutrients, from http://www.folikul.com/shen_min.pdf

55. Mori, H., Ohsawa, H., Tanaka, T. H., Taniwaki, E., Leisman, G., & Nishijo, K. (2004). Effect of massage on blood flow and muscle fatigue following isometric lumbar exercise. Medical Science Monitor, 10(5), CR173-178.

56. Georgala, S., Katoulis, A. C., Georgala, C., Moussatou, V., Bozi, E., & Stavrianeas, N. G. (2004). Topical estrogen therapy for androgenetic alopecia in menopausal females. Dermatology, 208(2), 178-179.

57. Abdel-Rahman, M. K. (2006). Effect of Pumpkin Seed (Cucurbita pepo L.) Diets on Benign Prostatic Hyperplasia (BPH): Chemical and Morphometric Evaluation in Rats. World Journal of Chemistry, 1(1), 33-40.

58. Winiarska, A., Mandt, N., Kamp, H., Hossini, A., Seltmann, H., Zouboulis, C. C., & Blume-Peytavi, U. (2006). Effect of 5alpha-Dihydrotestosterone and Testosterone on Apoptosis in Human Dermal Papilla Cells. Skin Pharmacology and Physiology, 19, 311-321. doi: 10.1159/000095251

59. Arck, P. C., Handjiski, B., Peters, E. M., et al. (2003). Stress inhibits hair growth in mice by induction of premature catagen development and deleterious perifollicular inflammatory events

via neuropeptide substance P-dependent pathways. American Journal of Pathology, 162(3), 803-814.

60. Bergfeld, W., & Harrison, S. (2009). Diffuse hair loss: Its triggers and management Cleveland Clinic Journal of Medicine, June 2009 vol. 76 6 361-367

61. Che-Jung Chang, Katie M. O'Brien, Alexander P. Keil, Symielle A. Gaston, Chandra L. Jackson, Dale P. Sandler, Alexandra J. White. (2022). Use of Straighteners and Other Hair Products and Incident Uterine Cancer. Journal of the National Cancer Institute DOI: https://doi.org/10.1093/jnci/djac165

62. Light, D.L., & Qian, W. (2022). Valisure Citizen Petition on Benzene in Dry Shampoo Products, October 31, 2022 www.valisure.com

63. Zhang Y, Birmann BM, Han J, et al. Personal use of permanent hair dyes and cancer risk and mortality in US women: prospective cohort study. BMJ.2020:m2942. doi:101136/bmj.m2942

Connect with Me Online:

Instagram: @LushLongHairCare

Facebook: www.facebook.com/LushLongHairCareGuide

www.ingramcontent.com/pod-product-compliance
Lightning Source LLC
Chambersburg PA
CBHW041300040426
42334CB00028BA/3102